Incision
Decisions

Incision Decisions

A GUIDE TO GETTING THROUGH SURGERY, RECOVERY, AND YOUR HOSPITAL STAY

◆ ◆ ◆

Kaye Newton

ISBN: 0692832548
ISBN 13: 9780692832547
Library of Congress Control Number: 2017932037
Linland Press
North Charleston, South Carolina

For my family

Table of Contents

Introduction

◆ ◆ ◆

PLANNING FOR SURGERY AND RECOVERY can be daunting. The good news is that there are many simple, practical things you can do to prepare well. Educating yourself about your operation and recuperation process is a great first step. It will make you feel more in control and enable you to make better decisions about your medical care.

Like you, I had questions before my first major surgery, which had a six-week recovery period with lifting and driving restrictions. Here are some of the things I wondered about:

- How do I find a good hospital and surgeon?
- How will my family eat if I can't drive to the grocery store or cook for five weeks after my operation?
- How much information do I tell my boss about my upcoming surgery?
- Who will do my laundry, since I will not be allowed to bend at the waist or lift more than five pounds?
- If I can't lean over for six weeks, how will I shave my fast-growing leg hair?

I spent too much time focused on the last question, when, in retrospect, I needed to deal with the other four questions. But to distract myself from my anxiety, I fixated on minor issues like body-hair management. Once I checked into the hospital, I faced reality. I would be out of commission for six weeks. Who would take care of my three active kids, household chores, part-time job, and emotionally needy dog? I needed help and a plan! I scribbled my first recovery plan, tracking offers of meals and rides, on a World Wildlife Fund calendar. Next to photos of depressed penguins, I drew squiggly lines linking appointments and kids' activities to offers of help.

Four months later, I went in for another unexpected major surgery with a six-week recovery. By this time I knew, before checking into the hospital, to send my dog and kids to my in-laws, freeze six meat loaves, and purchase a bottle of Nair with a four-foot spray capacity. I also drafted a surgery and recovery plan, which was the starting point of this book. (Since I was losing organs at a rapid rate, I wanted to document what I had learned in case this trend continued.) Eight months later, my eleven-year-old son had an emergency operation to repair his broken elbow and arm. Since I understood basic "hospitalese," the strange medical jargon spoken by doctors, I could comfort him by explaining medical terms and procedures.

The suggestions and advice in this book are based on issues that came up during my surgical experiences and family members' operations, as well as discussions with medical professionals and fellow patients and reviews of accredited hospital websites. It's information I wish I had known *before* my first operation. Studies indicate that people have better surgical outcomes when they are prepared for their upcoming operations.[1] By opening this book, you are already taking a positive step in educating yourself.

I Need Surgery?!

Like most normal people, I avoid hospitals. In fact, I would rather stay in the *Poltergeist* house, in the room with the clown, than check into a medical facility. Even the scent of a hospital, that mix of disinfectant spray and lime Jell-O, spooks me. Because of my medical-facility phobia, I did everything I possibly could to avoid having a hysterectomy, my first major surgery. I tried over- and under-the-counter medicine, exercises, outpatient medical procedures, acupuncture, and Chinese medicine. But these remedies failed. I ended up having a medical emergency, a hospitalization, and a life-saving operation with a six-week recovery.

To my surprise, my hospital stay was very tolerable. (My presurgery anxiety was worse than my actual operation.) And because of my surgery, I'm still here, with a much better quality of life. There are times when you need a knee replaced, a heart fixed, or a bone mended so you can keep on truckin'. **One of the best things you can do for your health is to be actively involved in your medical care.** This includes understanding what is involved in the weeks leading up to your surgery and what you will need to do during the recovery process.

The first step in getting ready for surgery is to select a good surgeon. Often your primary-care doctor, who may be your internist or family practitioner, is the person who suggests that you need an operation. He or she may refer you to one or more surgeons. Then it's up to you to decide who will perform your surgery.

CHAPTER 1

Finding the Best Surgeon to Perform Your Operation

Surgeons are usually confident, directive perfectionists. (As preschoolers, they likely corrected their Mommy and Me teachers and were the self-appointed kings of four square.) Surgeons need to be self-assured and decisive, since they are running the operating room and making important life-altering decisions.

But you also want to be confident in your surgeon. Ideally, you want a surgeon who has the following qualities.

Seven Qualities You Want in Your Surgeon

- Is board certified. A doctor who is board certified has passed state medical exams and is also committed to keeping current with the latest medical advancements and best practices in his or her specialty.[1]
- Specializes in your type of surgery. The more complex and difficult the surgery, the more you need a highly specialized expert.

- Performs your surgery on a regular basis and has performed the surgery for at least several years. (There is a reason the adage "practice makes perfect" exists.)
- Has low complication rates and high surgery success rates. You can ask the surgeon for this information.
- Is recommended by other medical professionals or family or friends
- Accepts your insurance
- Operates at a large, well-regarded, accredited hospital.

Where do you find this star surgeon?

Start by asking your internal medicine and family doctors, "If I were your sister/brother/partner and needed this surgery, who would you recommend?" Then branch out to friends and family members in the medical profession and see if they can suggest a surgeon. You can also approach people who have had your operation. Use social networks like Facebook, Nextdoor.com, and your e-mail contacts to ask for recommendations. Often the same doctors' names will pop up. Pick the name that is recommended often, and call to see if the doctor accepts your insurance.

Hospital employees can be a great source of recommendations. An emergency room (ER) doctor who examined me at three in the morning gave me an excellent surgeon recommendation. You could call a medical group and ask to speak to a nurse who works in the area of surgery you need. Explain your situation and ask the nurse whom she recommends. If she responds that all the surgeons are good, ask for specifics. Is one of the doctors using a new surgical technique? Did any of the surgeons just complete medical training? (You want a surgeon who has several years of experience performing your surgery.)

For a very complex surgery, you might want to consider traveling to an expert surgeon at a large medical center. To find this expert surgeon, you need to do some research. For example, if you need a specialized heart surgeon, you could access the *US News and World Report* "Best Hospitals" national rankings online and see the best hospitals for heart surgery. Let's say the Cleveland Clinic and Mayo Clinic are highly ranked. You could go to their websites and look for the doctors who perform your specific surgery. You can then call those surgeons' offices and ask the nurses for doctor recommendations and see if they take your insurance. You could also type the surgeons' names into PubMed.gov to determine if they have published recent medical research. The doctors who publish research are usually experts in their field. PubMed.gov contains thousands of articles on unpronounceable medical topics. I just try to focus on finding doctors' names.

While I glanced at the online doctor-rating sites, I kept in mind that unhappy patients are more apt to rate their physicians. The majority of people like their surgeons but don't bother to review them. I did look to see if my surgeons were board certified, if they specialized in my operation, where they trained and worked, and if they had done research on my condition.

Scheduling a Surgical Appointment

Since an initial surgical consultation usually takes more time than a routine office visit, mention to the scheduler that you might need surgery. Try to schedule the appointment first thing in the morning, before doctors get swamped and behind in their schedules. Ask about any medical tests and information you will need to bring with you, and find out if the surgeon takes your insurance.

For one of my surgeries, there were two equally qualified doctors, but one was booked for weeks. I wanted surgery as soon as possible, so I made an appointment with the doctor who had availability. If your selected surgeon is booked solid, you can call repeatedly in case there is a cancellation, or ask your primary-care doctor to call the surgeon to see if she can squeeze you into her schedule. If you have a friend or family member with a personal connection to the doctor, he or she might be able to get you an appointment.

How to Prepare for Meeting with a Surgeon for the First Time

During your first meeting, the surgeon will review your medical tests and reports and probably give you a physical exam. Be sure to bring your medical information with you or have your current doctor send it to the surgeon. You might want to call to make sure that the surgeon's office has received your file before your appointment.

Also, do some basic research on your surgery so you understand what the doctor is saying. You don't need to become a medical expert, but it helps to have general knowledge of your potential operation. Surgeons want you to be well informed and aware of the outcomes of an operation. You are a key participant in the surgical process.

For information on surgeries, you could type your operation into the following websites:

- MedlinePlus (http://medlineplus.gov), the National Institutes of Health website for patients and families
- Mayo Clinic (https://www.mayoclinic.org)
- University of California, San Francisco, Medical Center (https://www.ucsfhealth.org)

Bring a list of questions for the surgeon to the appointment.

QUESTIONS YOU SHOULD ASK A SURGEON

* Do I really need this surgery? How will this surgery help me? Will the benefits from this operation be long-term?
* What are the alternatives to surgery? What will happen to me if I don't do this surgery?
* What type of operation do you recommend for me? Is this the newest surgical technique? Can my operation be done as a minimally invasive surgery? (In general, minimally invasive surgery is associated with less pain and fewer complications than traditional open surgery.[2])
* How many of these surgeries do you do and what are your outcomes? How does this compare to your peers?
* What complications are associated with this surgery? How common are they? Am I at particular risk for any of these complications?
* Could you tell me about your typical patients' recovery process? Do you think my recovery will be typical? How long will I be out of commission?
* Could I talk to some of your former patients who had this surgery?
* Do I need this surgery immediately? If I decide to wait on it, what are the consequences?

It's a good idea to bring an attentive friend or family member to surgical appointments when you are getting a lot of information. He or she can take notes and ask questions. For minor or routine appointments, I didn't feel like I needed the support. However, during major surgical consultations, my brain froze at the word "incision." I tuned out important information and listened in on conversations in the hallway or looked down at my doctor's surprisingly stylish footwear. While the doctor explained her complex surgical techniques, I nodded along and thought, "Those are *cute* strappy sandals. But they are high. How does she race down the hospital corridor for a code blue without breaking her neck or snapping a three-inch heel?" As the surgeon pointed to a detailed diagram of the female anatomy, I bobbed my head and wondered, "Did I see those shoes at that good TJ Maxx? Next to the piles of lobster wall décor, deep in a cart of Spanx for men?" Since I was mentally miles away, shoe hunting through shaping briefs, I was fortunate to have a family member listening closely to the doctor and taking notes.

If you don't have anyone to come to your consultation, you could ask the doctor if you can record the appointment. This is easy to do with a smartphone, but you need to get permission ahead of time. Some doctors are comfortable with being taped, while others have policies against it.

What Is My Doctor Saying? Understanding Medical Jargon

Surgeons have spoken medical jargon, also known as "hospitalese," for years. Occasionally they forget that patients might not understand complex, hard-to-pronounce medical terms based on Latin and Greek roots. Since the average patient is not fluent in hospitalese, confusion can result.

On one occasion, a surgeon casually mentioned that he could give me a "robotic bilateral salpingo-oophorectomy using a laparoscope."

While his tone suggested that this would be as easy as a nail trim, I panicked and my brain screeched, "ROBOTS ARE GOING TO CUT OUT MY DOODAD-THINGAMAJIGGY USING A WATCHAMACALLIT-SCOPE?!" I interrupted the doctor to ask him to speak in simple English. (It can be helpful to request that your surgeon explain things as if you are his slightly demented elderly aunt or Forrest Gump.) Once I understood what the doctor was saying, I repeated my interpretation of his words back to him, and he corrected me as needed.

Occasionally, doctors draw pictures, which make things clearer. Sometimes they'll review a pamphlet about your condition. Take notes and circle important items on the handouts. Ask whom you should call if you have additional questions. You are not "bothering" your doctor or nurse when you have questions that you need answered. Doctors and nurses chose their professions because they truly wanted to help people. While they are busy individuals, they want you to understand your medical situation and their recommendations.

There is a basic guide to medical jargon at the back of this book. It translates medical terms like "rhinorrhea" into regular words like "runny nose." You can also look up medical words in an online health dictionary at Medlineplus.gov or the websites of prominent teaching hospitals, such as the Mayo Clinic.

UNDERSTANDING COMPLICATIONS

Your surgeon will describe the risks associated with your operation. Every operation has the potential for complications. If your upcoming surgery is elective or cosmetic, it makes sense to understand and carefully weigh the risk of complications against the potential benefits of the surgery. In general, complications can arise from things like infections or blood loss and can prolong a hospital stay. Your medical team will answer your questions about the nature and frequency of the complications associated with your specific operation.

If you need surgery to stay alive, such as a kidney transplant or a quadruple heart bypass, you may not need an in-depth review of potential complications. You are having the surgery no matter what. Pick the best surgeon who specializes in your procedure and operates at a highly ranked hospital. (Highly ranked hospitals usually have well-run intensive care units [ICUs] if something goes wrong.) Researching every potential complication associated with your operation can be unsettling. Why "borrow worry" about something that may never happen? Preparing for surgery is a more productive way to spend your time. If a complication occurs, your medical team can deal with it. Hospital staffs address complications on a daily basis.

WHAT IF MY SURGEON DOESN'T HAVE A SPARKLING PERSONALITY?

While it's nice to have a surgeon with a wonderful bedside manner, I wanted the most technically skilled doctor who specialized in my type of operation. Unlike my pediatrician or general practitioner, I wasn't planning on seeing my surgeon on a regular basis. I'd be unconscious for the three-and-half-hour surgery and self-medicated for the half-hour post-op appointment. While I needed to understand my doctor's plan and have my questions answered, it wasn't necessary for my surgeon to have a scintillating personality. She wasn't joining my book club or meeting me for mimosas to catch up on our weekend shenanigans. Successful surgeries depend on the doctor's hand skills, good judgment, technical training, and experience.

Participating in Your Surgical Plan

Doctors often want your participation in a surgical plan. For certain operations, your doctor will ask you to make a decision or state a preference. You may have input regarding the type of anesthesia to be used (local or general) or what type of implant you want. For example, when preparing for a hip replacement, you could be asked if you prefer porcelain or titanium. When this first comes up, you might think, "Why in the world is my surgeon talking to me about cookware? Or is he referring to toilet bowls?" The surgeon is giving you a choice about the material of your new hip. He will explain the pros and cons of the different types of hip implants, which can be made out of porcelain, metal, or plastic. Your surgeon can recommend which type is best for you, but you may get to decide which material you would like.

Occasionally, patients add another operation to their surgical plan. For example, someone might ask for a tummy tuck while going in for a hernia repair or request that weird skin tags are removed while doing a knee replacement. The advantage of undergoing two procedures at one time is that you check into the hospital and have anesthesia only once. The downside is that the surgery time and recovery period with an added operation could be longer and have a higher rate of complications. If you are interested in an additional operation, your medical team can advise you about the associated pros and cons.

How to Get a Second Opinion

After hearing the doctor's surgical plan, it's a good idea to get a second opinion. This means asking another doctor to review your original doctor's evaluation of your condition. A second opinion can confirm your original doctor's recommendations or offer a new perspective on your medical situation. Each doctor will have his or her own approach to surgery, so you'll learn something from each meeting. It's worth the time and effort to talk to at least two surgeons about your operation.

I don't like to hurt people's feelings, and I worried, unnecessarily, that I would upset my original well-qualified surgeon by asking for a second opinion. Would she think I didn't trust her judgment and recommendations? Was I cheating on her by consulting with another doctor behind her back? Not at all! Physicians often expect patients to get a second opinion about major surgery. Most insurance companies pay for second opinions, and some even require them. Contact your insurance company to see what your policy covers.

The second doctor will need to see your medical records, lab and test results, x-rays, and physician reports. Your original doctor's medical staff should be able to send this information to the second doctor after you sign a release form. Or you can get a full set of your medical information and bring it with you to your second-opinion appointment.

Surgeons often welcome the additional information from another physician's review of your case. Doctors like to learn from each other. But you may be unsure how to ask for a second opinion. Here are two ways to approach your doctor:

Doctor, I appreciate the information you have given me. I like to cover all the bases before making a major medical decision, and I would like to get a second opinion, just for reassurance. Could your staff send my files to Dr. Barry Woo at Cleveland Clinic?

My insurance company requires that I have a second opinion before they will pay for surgery. Could your staff send my files to Dr. Joan Lewis at St. John's Hospital?

If the two surgeons' opinions differ, you can go back to the original doctor and see if she can explain the differences to you. You could also ask a family member or friend who is in the medical profession to give input about the differing opinions, or consider getting a third surgeon's opinion.

CHAPTER 2

Gathering Information and Choosing the Right Hospital

◆ ◆ ◆

GATHERING INFORMATION ABOUT YOUR RECOVERY

THERE ARE PIECES OF INFORMATION you will need from your medical team before you create a plan to manage your work and household during your hospitalization and recovery. It was imperative for me to know the answers to these questions:

- When will I be allowed to drive again?
- How long until I can lift more than five pounds or lean over to do a load of laundry?
- When should I tell my boss I'll be back to work?
- Will I need a special diet or physical therapy after surgery?
- When can I shower after my operation?

Sometimes surgeons give noncommittal answers to these questions, such as, "If you listen to your body, you'll know when you're ready," or, "You can resume your activities as tolerated." Doctors say these things because people's bodies recover at different rates. If you get a noncommittal answer, you can reword the question using the **average patient approach**. For example, you can ask the following:

- When does your average patient resume driving after this type of surgery?
- When has your average patient gone back to work?
- At what point does your average patient safely lift five pounds?
- Do you consider me to be an average patient? Do I have any health conditions that would affect the length of my recovery?

You can also question the nurses when the doctor is out of earshot. (Nurses are chattier when the doctors are not around and can give you the inside scoop.) Find a way to communicate with your medical team that you are comfortable with, whether it's in person, over the phone, or by e-mail through a patient portal. It's also a good idea to ask the medical staff to recommend websites that explain your upcoming surgery. Then go to those recommended websites.

Do *Not* Use Dr. Google Randomly!

If you arbitrarily google your upcoming operation, you will learn about hideous surgery experiences that you will wish you never knew about. You will want to cancel your necessary operation and flee to an uninhabited tropical island where you can't even find a Band-Aid. People who have problems with their surgery rant online, often in multiple forums. The majority of surgeries go well. The silent majority won't write anything on the Internet. They are too busy resting on their couches, popping OxyContin, and chuckling at Ellen's Dance Dare.

So stick to directive googling and go to websites that are recommended by your doctor or developed by surgeons and peer reviewed by physicians, such as the American Academy of Orthopaedic Surgeons' OrthoInfo. Also, respected medical centers like the University of California, Los Angeles, (UCLA) Medical Center and Johns Hopkins Hospital usually have reliable, up-to-date information on their sites.

Some hospitals offer surgery preparation workshops or online informational videos. My mom went to a hip-replacement class where she learned about presurgery exercises and what to expect during her recovery. The more information that you gather about your upcoming surgery, the better you can plan and prepare.

Picking a Good Hospital for Your Surgery

Once you pick your surgeon, she will tell you where she has hospital privileges, which means where she performs her operations. Some hospitals have better outcomes, patient satisfaction ratings, and lower infection rates than others. Certain hospitals are known for their successful heart surgeries, while others are cancer centers. You can check hospital ratings on sites and web pages like ConsumerReports.org, Medicare.gov's Hospital Compare, or *US News and World Report*'s health section. Ideally, you want a well-respected hospital that has positive ratings and where your operation is frequently performed. Ask your doctor which hospital has the best outcomes for your surgery and what she recommends. **If you have to drive farther to a better hospital, it can be worth the extra travel time.**[1]

If your insurance will only cover a stay at a so-so hospital, at least you are going in prepared to be extra vigilant. You can check in with a gallon of hand sanitizer, a tub of disinfectant wipes with bleach, and a highly proactive advocate by your side. Tips and suggestions for avoiding hospital-acquired infections and medical errors will be covered in later chapters.

Some hospitals are teaching hospitals, where new doctors, called residents, are trained. Residents have graduated from medical school and are part of patients' health-care teams. They are learning the ropes and work under the guidance of experienced physicians. When you first hear about residents, you might think, "Hmm, I am not sure if I want a brand-new doctor practicing on me. Could he possibly try out his skills on someone else?" But I learned that being a patient in a teaching hospital has advantages. The residents are smart, motivated, and very thorough. They ask a lot of questions and serve as an extra set of eyes and ears for their attending physician, who is the experienced doctor in charge of your care. In a teaching hospital, there is always a resident around in the middle of the night who can help you. Teaching hospitals usually have better-quality ratings than nonteaching hospitals and conduct medical research.[2] So the doctors and residents often know about the latest cutting-edge treatments.

OUTPATIENT VERSUS INPATIENT SURGERY: WHICH WILL I HAVE?

For inpatient surgery, you are admitted to the hospital and spend the night. Inpatient surgeries are usually more complex than outpatient surgeries and require postsurgical monitoring by medical professionals. Typically, they are more expensive than outpatient surgeries and require advanced pain management tools such as morphine pumps.

Outpatient surgery is also known as same-day or ambulatory surgery. Outpatients have surgery and then go home later that day. You need to have someone drive you home after the operation. And it's often recommended that someone stay with you for at least twenty-four hours after surgery. Outpatient surgery can be performed in a hospital or clinic or even a doctor's office. Check before your operation to make sure that the facility is accredited and has good outcomes.

According to the Brigham and Women's Hospital online health encyclopedia, advances in medical technology and pain management have enabled more surgeries to be performed as outpatient procedures, including tonsillectomies and gallbladder removals. Some of the advantages of outpatient surgery are lower cost, recovering in the comfort of your home, and reduced exposure to hospital-acquired infections. Outpatient surgeries don't typically have as many unexpected complications or emergencies, so your operation is more likely to happen as scheduled.[3]

Your health insurance, type of surgery, health status, and other factors will determine whether your procedure will be inpatient or outpatient. Ultimately it's up to your surgeon's judgment and whether you have a need for hospital care.

While the information in upcoming chapters focuses on preparing and recovering from inpatient hospital stays, the majority of them also apply to outpatient operations.

WILL HEALTH INSURANCE COVER MY SURGERY?

Most insurance plans will pay for operations that are considered "medically necessary." But keep in mind that even with covered surgeries, you will probably have copays and deductibles that will need to be met. Insurance companies usually don't pay for plastic surgery, unless it can be shown that you need the surgery to function. It's unlikely that a face-lift would be covered. But an insurance company might approve a nose job if you have difficulty breathing out of your current nose. For some operations, insurance companies have conditions that need to be met before they will pay for surgery. For example, in order for bariatric weight-loss surgery to be approved, insurance companies may require that you have a body mass index above forty.

Before committing to surgery, call your insurance company to see how much it will pay for your operation. (If you are over sixty-five and have Medicare, call 800-MEDICARE or go to Medicare. gov.) You also need to know if your insurance plan requires prior authorization and if you must go to an in-network surgeon. If you go to an out-of-network doctor, you could end up with a staggering hospital bill. For highly specialized surgery, such as removing a brain tumor, there might not be a local in-network expert doctor who has the technical skills that your situation requires. In that case, you could call the best specialists around the country and see if they will take your insurance.

Doctors' offices constantly deal with insurance companies, and the staff is familiar with ways to get coverage and authorizations. If your insurance company denies coverage, contact your doctor's office. They may have tips on how you can appeal the insurance company's decision. An appeal often involves persistent letter writing from you and your doctor on why your surgery is medically necessary and should be covered.

SHOULD I CONSIDER TRAVELING TO HAVE SURGERY?

Usually, you can receive good medical care at a hospital near your home, and it's not worth the time and expense to travel for surgery. Most procedures can be handled by a large local hospital.[4] However, if you need a highly specialized surgery or don't live near a major city, you might want to think about traveling. There are highly ranked medical centers, like the Cleveland Clinic, where patients frequently travel five hundred miles or more to be treated. They offer hospital concierge services that coordinate flights, transportation from the airport, and hotel stays on their campus. Patients often stay for several days at a hotel after discharge from the hospital. When patients return home, their local doctors handle follow-up care.

Before you decide to travel for surgery, check if your insurance company will cover the operation at the distant hospital. Keep in mind that insurance does not usually pay for travel or a hotel room. So it can be expensive. Also, you will need to make sure that you get all your tests and medical information to bring back to your local doctor. And if you have a rare complication during your recovery, you might have to travel back to see the surgeon who did your operation.

PICKING YOUR SURGERY DATE AND TIME

One of my surgeries was a medical emergency, and I received the first available surgery slot. If your surgery is urgent, make sure you tell the scheduler that you need it ASAP. I based my other surgery dates on my doctor's availability, when my husband could take time off from work, and holidays and important family events. For example, I didn't want to miss Halloween, which my kids start planning for in July, and I wanted to be in decent shape for Christmas. So I picked a surgery date during the first week of November.

You may want to have knee- or hip-replacement surgery in the spring or summer to avoid crutches and canes sliding on winter ice. If you love swimming in the summer, you might schedule surgery in the fall, since doctors often instruct patients to avoid pools, hot tubs, and the ocean while incisions heal. Also, if you have met your high insurance deductible by October or have a medical-expense savings account with a use-it-or-lose-it provision, then you'll want to schedule surgery before the end of the year. Try to avoid surgery at a teaching hospital during July, when the new doctors begin their residencies.

It can be beneficial to schedule surgery on a Monday or a Tuesday, so a full medical staff is available during your hospital stay. (Some physical therapists and doctors don't work on weekends.) Since I would get "hangry" (a state of being angry when hungry), I scheduled surgery as early as possible in the morning. That way I didn't have to fast as long. (You typically can't eat or drink anything after midnight the day before surgery.) Also, surgery is like flying. If you fly later in the day, there is a stronger possibility of unexpected delays due to late connections. In the hospital, an emergency could come in or an earlier surgery could take longer than scheduled, and your operation could get bumped to a later time.

WHAT IF I NEED EMERGENCY SURGERY?

Surgery for appendicitis and some types of broken bones, like a hip fracture, may need to be performed as soon as possible. You might get the surgeon who is available to operate and on call. But when you are in the ER, ask the doctors for recommendations. The best specialist could be available in five hours, and it might be okay to wait for her. You can also call your primary-care doctor and ask if you are at the best hospital for your emergency surgery. If not, consider making a request to be transferred to a hospital that has the specialists you need.

For my son's elbow fracture, we went to a local ER, where the doctor took x-rays and said that my son needed surgery as soon as possible. But the ER doctor also told us that his hospital didn't have the expertise to operate on my son's elbow. He sent us to a local children's hospital, where a pediatric orthopedist did the surgery.

CHAPTER 3

Lining Up Help

◆ ◆ ◆

IT's IMPORTANT TO HAVE AN advocate in the hospital and help at home while recovering from surgery. How much help you need depends on the type of operation, your household dynamics, and how fast you heal. While many of us like to be self-reliant, surgery is a life event when we need assistance.

THE IMPORTANT ROLE OF YOUR ADVOCATE

Your advocate is the person who goes to the hospital with you to be your supporter and champion throughout your stay. Usually, it's a relative or close friend who is attentive, communicates well, and is willing to watch hours of hospital TV. (Hospital TV defaults to ninety-minute programs like "Hand Washing 101: How to Squirt Soap Accurately and Use a Paper Towel Instead of Your Germy Hospital Gown.")

Since you'll be groggy and bedbound after your operation, it's important to have an advocate there to remember the doctor's orders, speak up if anything doesn't seem right, and communicate with friends and family.

THE HOSPITAL ADVOCATE'S DUTIES INCLUDE THE FOLLOWING:

- Drive you to and from the hospital and stay in the hospital during surgery.
- Visit daily, especially on weekends and holidays when there might be reduced staff.
- Talk to the surgeon about the results of your operation.
- Update family and friends about your surgery.
- Communicate with hospital staff: assist you with ordering meals from the cafeteria and calling for a nurse when you first get out of bed.
- Question the doctors and nurses if something doesn't seem right.
- Speak up if the medical staff doesn't wash their hands before examining you or changing your intravenous (IV) line or catheter.
- Ask about the pills the nurses dole out. Ask about the medicines that are in your IV bag. What are they? What do they do?
- Make sure you stay hydrated and drink lots of water postsurgery.
- Manage your visitors. If your brother-in-law appears at your bedside with a whooping cough that he says is "just allergies," your advocate hands him a surgical mask or, even better, suggests that he visit you at home when you are both feeling well.
- Understand your discharge instructions and get your prescriptions filled.

WHAT IF I CAN'T FIND AN ADVOCATE TO BE WITH ME IN THE HOSPITAL?

Anyone who checks into a hospital, with or without an advocate, should be prepared to speak up if something doesn't seem right. Ask questions about your medicines and procedures. You can be your own advocate and follow the suggestions in the upcoming section on reducing medical errors.

If you don't have an advocate because of the amount of time the job requires, consider dividing the role among friends and family. Maybe a close work colleague could be your advocate for a Saturday afternoon, and a cousin could take a shift the next day. If an advocate can only come in for a few hours, ask her to be with you during discharge, when you are receiving a lot of information and need a ride home.[1] It's also helpful to have an advocate right after surgery, when you are heavily drugged and might be unable to speak up for yourself.

Another option would be to bring in your own private-duty nurse or paid companion. This can be expensive, since it's not covered by insurance. You can ask your doctor about the hospital's staffing and if she thinks hiring a nurse is something to consider. It might depend on whether the hospital has a good nurse-to-patient ratio, the type of operation you are having, and your overall health.

Your regular hospital nurses can be advocates for you. Let them know if you are on your own. While it's always important to be respectful and pleasant to your nurses, you might want to up the ante and bring wrapped chocolates or other treats to share with the staff.

DETERMINING HOW MUCH HELP YOU WILL NEED

The first week postsurgery is the hardest. You will be on pain medicine and resting with your feet up for a large part of the day. It's great if your advocate or any responsible person can stay with you after you leave the hospital. He or she can pick up groceries, do laundry, drive the kids to activities, walk the dog, and provide meals. Your helper could stock the fridge before leaving and wipe down the kitchen counters.

Try to plan what type of assistance you will need after your helper departs. Look at your calendar and make a list of all your needs and wants during your recovery. Then postpone your wants and anything thing else that can wait. Keep in mind that it's better to schedule too much help than to have too little. If you are feeling great after surgery, you can always cancel the meals and support.

I was told there could be no bending, vacuuming, lifting anything over five pounds, or pushing a grocery cart for at least six weeks after my first operation. And no driving until I was completely off my prescription pain meds. The chart below gives you an idea of how I tried to manage my household and part-time job during my recovery period. (There is a blank copy of this chart in the appendix at the back of the book for your use.)

EXAMPLE OF A SIX-WEEK-RECOVERY COVERAGE CHECKLIST

What Needs to Be Covered	Specific Action
Caring for the kids and pets while I'm in the hospital	Ask mother-in-law or close friend.
Shopping for groceries	Order online and have groceries delivered. Or ask a friend to pick up groceries.

Preparing meals	Organizer will ask friends to bring meals on Tuesdays and Thursdays for one month. Start meals one week after surgery when husband goes back to work. Pick up or order in weekend meals.
Getting a ride to post-op doctor's appointment	Ask mother-in-law or close friend for ride.
Picking up prescriptions from pharmacy	Find a pharmacy that delivers or ask a friend to pick up.
Paying bills	Pay bills before surgery.
Doing laundry	Instruct kids on how to do the laundry.
Running dishwasher and putting dishes away	Kids will do, or buy disposable paper plates and paper cups.
Managing work	Let boss and HR know leave-of-absence dates.
Vacuuming and cleaning house	Let it go.
Feeding and walking dog	Kids will handle the dog.
Getting kids to their activities and friends' birthday parties	Ask organizer to find someone to drive kids.

Hiring a neighborhood middle schooler to help with kids and dogs while I am home recovering	Ask organizer to find someone or post on Nextdoor.com, my neighborhood website.
Getting teeth cleaned at dentist's office	Postpone.
Volunteering at PTO book fair	Cancel.
Doing yard work	Ignore.
Making dinner reservations, having lunches out, and going to concerts	Postpone or cancel.
Getting a pedicure	Postpone.
Going on Thanksgiving trip to see family	Cancel and plan to go later in the year.

TELLING PEOPLE (OR NOT) ABOUT YOUR UPCOMING SURGERY

Your upcoming surgery is part of your private health information, and whom you tell about it is entirely up to you; it might depend on the type of operation you are having and how much help you need. I told my immediate family, close friends, my kids' teachers, and my boss about my surgeries. I needed and appreciated their support. But I didn't tell my hair stylist, distant relatives, or veterinarian. There were many times when I didn't want to think about or discuss my health issues, so I only mentioned my surgery to those people I felt needed to know.

I communicated the news of my operation via text or e-mail after I had passed the prescreening tests and had a definite plan in place. That way I could let friends know how many days I would be in the hospital and when I would be home. When I had an unexpected hospitalization, my husband asked two close friends to discreetly round up helpers to take my kids until I was back on my feet.

When asking for time off from work, it's up to you to decide how much information you want to reveal. You can simply say, "I need six weeks off for major surgery," or you can get into the specifics of your operation. It depends on your relationship with your boss and what you are comfortable divulging.

Friends who wanted to share their surgeries with a large group utilized social media like Facebook and CaringBridge.org. On CaringBridge, patients can explain their operations, give health updates, and receive messages from friends and family. If you have a newly diagnosed serious illness and upcoming surgery, it can be overwhelming to send and receive multiple phone calls, e-mails, and texts. You might want to ask your organizer if he or she could create a Facebook page or CaringBridge site, which is easy to use and enables everyone to receive updates on your health at the same time. You can then focus on going to doctors' appointments and preparing for surgery.

APPOINTING AN ORGANIZER TO COMMUNICATE YOUR NEEDS AND GATHER HELP

Your organizer is the point person who lines up your meals, transportation, and other needs. He or she can let everyone know if you need more food and what your health status is. The organizer will redirect offers of assistance and say things like "Please don't make your lima-bean casserole for the Newtons. They have enough meals. How about driving Kaye's kids to soccer practice on Tuesday?" Your organizer can also be a gatekeeper. If you aren't up for visitors, let the organizer know and she can communicate that.

The organizer can use e-mail, texts, and free websites like Lotsahelpinghands.com, Mealtrain.com, and Takethemameal.com to manage meals and your needs. Usually, the organizer is a good friend who will come forward and offer to help. If no one steps up, your spouse can be the organizer, or he can ask a friend or family member to take charge.

Use Caregiving Websites to Organize Meals, Rides, and Other Help

Free caregiving websites like Lotsahelpinghands.com simplify the process of setting up support. Instead of scrolling through multiple texts and e-mail offers of assistance, you and your organizer can easily set up a "community" (a list of your friends' and families' e-mail addresses). You list what type of meals and rides you need on a shared calendar and then send out links to it. Friends and family click on the link and sign up to help. Lotsa Helping Hands sends meal reminders and has sections for health announcements and get-well messages.

My meal schedule was created on a free website called Takethemameal.com. The meals and casseroles were delicious and the size of sofa cushions, so we ate them for two consecutive dinners. We left a big cooler by our front door. Friends dropped off food in the cooler when I was napping or resting.

Here's what my meal plan on Takethemameal.com looked like:

Meals for: Kaye Newton
Meal coordinator info: Jane Organizer: cell 222-222-2222
Deliver meals to: Kaye's house, 100 Recovery Lane

Notes from meal coordinator:
Let's help the Newton family while Kaye is recovering from sur-gery. They appreciate your offer to make a dinner!

Please drop off your meal between 5:00 and 6:00 p.m. in the cooler by the front door. The family does not have any allergies and enjoys any type of food. Please send food in containers that do not need to be returned. Takeout meals from a local restaurant are great too. You can text Kaye at 333-333-3333 with any additional information about your meal.

Kaye's mother will be staying November 11–13, so please include food for an extra adult during those days.

Meal plan on Takethemameal.com		
Date	Meal Provider	What I Plan to Bring
Tuesday, November 11	Laney Koon	Chicken soup and rolls, cookies
Thursday, November 13	Veronica Robin	Pork loin and potatoes
Tuesday, November 18	Lori Dunn	Thai or Chinese takeout
Thursday, November 20	Courtney Ripley	Zoe's chicken kabobs
Tuesday, November 25	Suzanne Moore	Lasagna
Thursday, November 27	Alix Foster	Layered pasta casserole
Tuesday, December 2	Rachael Sam	To be determined
Thursday, December 4	Patti Berry-Kaffke	Lasagna roll-ups
Tuesday, December 9	Natalie Latham	Taco twist casserole

Asking for Help: How to Do It and How to Redirect Offers

"Let me know if I can do anything."

You will hear this kind, vague offer dozens of times before your upcoming surgery. People like to be helpful. They are sincere when they offer assistance. They just don't know what you need. Turn their thoughtful offers into specific beneficial actions. Give them the opportunity to feel good. Once you've recovered, you can pay the favor forward by helping someone else.

The following are examples of responses to a general offer of help.

> *Nice person: "I heard that you are having surgery. Please let me know if I can do anything."*

> *You: "Thanks! I'll give your name to Jane, who is organizing meals for me."*

Then send a quick text or e-mail and have Jane put the person on the list to make you a meal.

> *You: "Thank you! I'm not sure how my Lenny is going to get to baseball practice next week when I can't drive. Any chance you could give him a ride to Thursday's practice?"*

> *You: "A playdate for my kids would be great. They are going to be stir-crazy in the house while I can't drive. Could they go home with your daughter next Thursday after school?"*

If you don't want to give these responses, you can say, "Thanks. Jane, my organizer, can let you know when I need help." And then make sure to tell Jane about the offer.

Other ways to ask for help could be by sending a group e-mail or text or posting a general statement on your Facebook page or other social media:

Thanks for your offers of help. We appreciate it. Jane, the organizer, is coordinating meals and rides for my kids. You can contact Jane on her cell, 222-222-2222, or e-mail Jane12@gmail.com, and she can let you know what we need.

CREATE AN INFORMATION MEMO FOR CARETAKERS

If someone is coming from out of town to take care of you and your family, it's helpful to write down information about your household. This memo would be similar to what you would give a babysitter or house sitter if you were going on a two-week trip to the Caribbean, instead of a "recovercation" on your couch.

You could include the following:

* Contact information for your organizer, close friends, and neighbors (in case your caretaker gets locked out of the house or needs help if your dog runs away), veterinarian, pediatrician, and doctors' offices
* Codes and passwords for things like alarm systems, voice mail, e-mail, and Netflix
* Locations of grocery stores, pharmacy, kids' schools, and kids' activities

- Links to your meal schedule and other offers of help
- Kids' schedules—list who needs to go where and when and which friends are giving them rides to school and extracurricular actives. You might want to include suggested bedtimes and what time they need to get ready for school.
- If family members are on medications, list when they should take them. If anyone has a food allergy, list who can eat what.

GETTING THROUGH YOUR RECOVERY ON YOUR OWN WITHOUT HELPERS

There are three keys to getting through recovery on your own. The first is to be as prepared as possible. Before you check into the hospital, make sure you understand your postoperative restrictions. Ask when you can drive again, how much you can lift, and how often you can use the stairs. Find out if you will need crutches or a walker, and take them out for a test drive before surgery. Stock up on daily necessities and easy-to-open snacks, drinks, and frozen dinners. Do extra laundry and clean the house before surgery. Arrange your room and bed so that you have nearby water, snacks, a laptop, books, and a pad to write down when you take your medication. Make sure you have plenty of extra-strength Tylenol, and see the upcoming chapters for more details on preparing for your recovery.

The second key to recovering on your own is to utilize meal, grocery, and pharmacy delivery services. If you have lifting restrictions, ask that heavy items be distributed among several bags. Also, remember to wear a jacket or top with pockets so you can keep your charged cell phone with you. That way, you can easily call for a delivery or reach your doctor's office.

The third key is to outsource chores. Consider hiring housecleaners to help with laundry and vacuuming. If you have an active pet, board him in a kennel or get a pet sitter to come in and help during the first week of recovery. Also, many churches and synagogues have hospitality committees that enjoy providing free assistance and rides for people in their community. Uber or Lyft could get you to appointments. As a backup plan, get the number of a private nursing company that could come out to help if needed. (Check to see if your insurance company would cover this.) Finally, tell your doctor that you are going to be on your own, and she might suggest other means of support.

For the tech savvy, Google Home or Amazon Echo, virtual personal assistants, can be helpful during recovery. These devices, which retail between $130 and $180, obey voice commands and hook up to smart home appliances and the Internet. While resting in bed, you can call out, "Alexa," (the name of the Echo personal assistant) "turn on the lights and order a pepperoni pizza for dinner. Alexa, arrange an Uber pickup for Thursday and remind me to take my medicine every four hours." While you remain between the sheets issuing orders, Alexa willingly executes your list of instructions. (No sighing or grumbling from your robot friend. She is just "happy to help.") She can keep a list of questions for your doctor and calmly dial for assistance if you need it.

For someone living alone, it may be helpful to go from the hospital to a skilled nursing facility or rehabilitation facility. After my mom's knee-replacement surgery, she spent a week at a rehab facility, where she received meals, nursing care, and physical therapy twice a day. She also visited with therapy dogs and attended tai chi classes to improve her balance. By the time she came home, she was a week further along in her recovery and able to do more things for herself.

CHAPTER 4

Organizing Your Health Information and Paying for Surgery

◆ ◆ ◆

Why It's Important to Create a Central Repository for All Your Medical Information

You will get test results, pamphlets, and insurance bills from different doctors and from the hospital. Some of this information will be stored in electronic medical records that you can access online through a patient-portal account. But some information will come to you as hard copy, such as second opinions or genetic testing. *You* need to be the central repository of your medical information and be able to share it with your doctors. (Some doctors' offices are not yet electronically linked with each other.)

In order to get a full picture of your health and be your own advocate, you can keep all of your medical information in a central place using either a big paper-based medical binder or an electronic personal heath record.

Creating a big medical binder or an electronic personal health record will enable you to do the following:

* Make sure all your doctors have your updated medical information. Doctors may not have access to every test result or prescription. Take your binder or personal health record to appointments. That way, you can make sure your surgeon knows things like the results of the latest tests that your internist ordered.
* Learn more about your health. By reading things like magnetic resonance imaging (MRI) results and asking questions, you'll get a clearer picture of your health. The more informed you are, the better decisions you'll be able to make.
* Make sure that what needs to get done actually gets done. You can double-check that things such as the lab tests your specialist ordered were completed.

How to Make a Big Medical Binder for All Your Health Information

1. Buy a big three-ring binder, one stack of filler paper, dividers (some with pockets), tape, and a three-hole punch.
2. Gather your medical paperwork. Ask for copies of test results and reports over the phone or at appointments. Print out your electronic medical records, which can include doctors' notes, blood-pressure readings, and medical test results. You can access your electronic medical records from your online patient portal.
3. Type up a **health summary**, which lists these items:
    * *All* the medications and supplements you currently take or just stopped taking, including prescription drugs, over-the-counter drugs, vitamins, and herbal remedies. Include the amount you take and why you take it.
    * Allergies.

- Reactions you have had to medicines, anesthesia, or dyes used in tests like an MRI.
- Diseases, surgeries, or major illnesses you currently have or have had.
- Any serious health conditions that your immediate family has.

Make copies of this sheet so that you can hand it to your nurses and doctors or refer to it when filling out patient questionnaires. Save it on your computer so you can update it.

4. Organize your binder. I made tabs for each medical issue and put the related paperwork in chronological order. Also, some medical expenses might be tax-deductible, so it's a good idea to add a tab to keep track of them. If you have a living will or advance medical directive, make a tab and add it to the binder.

5. Get a business card from each doctor, nurse, physical therapist, and other medical professional you meet. Often they will hand a card to you, or you can find their cards at the front desk. Tape the cards on a sheet at the front of your binder for quick reference. Also, write down hints to your patient-portal password and username.

6. Create an **encouragement page** of pictures and quotes to comfort and motivate you through your medical journey. This could include pictures of your loved ones, drawings, magazine photos of a trip you want to take after surgery, or a quote, like one frequently attributed to Winston Churchill: "Never, never, never give up!" You could write down your own original inspirational thoughts. I scribbled a reminder that I been toughened up by past hardships and wrote: "I have survived a) a twenty-eight-hour labor, b) a housewide flying ant invasion while hosting company,

and c) fountain hairdos and culottes, which I wore from fifth to seventh grade. I got through these tough times, and I will get through surgery too!"

7. Use the binder when preparing for medical appointments. Write down questions you have for the doctor. List your most important questions first to make sure they are addressed. Keep medical articles, pamphlets, and research that you want to discuss with your doctor.

Put the binder somewhere you can find it. Take it with you to medical appointments. Write notes in it during discussions with doctors. Document follow-up items that you need to do after appointments or tests. If you review your notes and don't understand something the doctor said, call the nurse to clarify or e-mail the doctor directly through a patient portal.

Creating a Personal Health Record

If you don't want to make a big paper-based medical binder, you can create an electronic personal health record (PHR), which is a collection of your medical information that is stored on your computer or on the web. You can access your PHR through your phone, tablet, or computer. As with the big medical binder, you can decide what personal health information you want to put in your PHR, such as allergies, medications, health conditions, major surgeries, and your living will. Some PHRs help you track doctor appointments and health goals, like lowering your cholesterol, and can upload and analyze data from home monitoring devices like blood-pressure readings.[1]

You can create your own PHR, or you might be offered one by your hospital, doctors, insurer, or a commercial supplier. Some of these are free, and others charge a fee. Each supplier has its own application design and data-storage policies. You will need to determine which system is easiest for you to use and meets your data and privacy needs. For more information on how to create a PHR, see MyPHR.com, which is sponsored by the American Health Information Management Foundation.

While you are in charge of your PHR, keep in mind that a PHR is *not* the same as an electronic health record, which is created and updated by medical professionals.

A Brief Overview of Your Electronic Health Records

An electronic health record (EHR) is a digital collection of all your health history, including allergies, medications, lab tests, and notes from the doctors you have seen. If your internist orders a lab test or puts you on a new drug, it can be seen by your dermatologist and heart doctor via their tablets if their computer systems are connected. But not all doctors and hospitals are electronically linked. The medical field is working on this.

When you see a nurse or doctor, she will ask you a question and rapidly type your answer into a laptop or tablet. While you reveal your intimate health issues, your medical professional stares deeply into her computer screen or searches for the backspace key. As the nurse endlessly clicks her mouse, you might wonder if she is charting your health since birth or playing a long game of Tetris. But do not take her lack of eye contact personally; keep in mind that doctors and nurses are *required* by insurance companies and policy makers to accurately record and code oodles of medical information in an

EHR. They find this process frustrating and would much rather spend time interacting with patients than typing. But they need to input the information correctly to meet regulatory standards and so your insurance company will pay for your appointment, test, or procedure.

Electronic medical records can help doctors avoid ordering the same test or prescribing drugs that interact with each other. You can usually look at your EHR on a computer through a secure portal and see test results and review doctors' notes about your medical issues. Some patient portals allow you to send e-mails to your medical team and set up appointments.

EHRs and all medical information are protected by federal HIPAA (Health Insurance Portability and Accountability Act) privacy laws, and only certain specified individuals are permitted to see your health records. Medical staff members usually sign confidentiality agreements. If they break them, they can be fired and possibly sued. Doctors and hospitals also have computerized security safeguards to keep health information private.

Paying for Your Surgery

Three days before my surgery, I met with a hospital financial counselor as the first part of my preadmission appointment. The financial counselor wanted a copy of my insurance card and my personal information. She typed away and then revealed the estimated cost of my surgery and hospital stay. (I should have braced myself for this number. Or at least been offered nitrous oxide or a Xanax.) The estimated gross cost of my hysterectomy and one-night hospital stay was $36,000. Since we didn't have $36,000 to spend on surgery and one night in the hospital,

I stopped stressing about going under the knife and started worrying about selling my worn minivan to pay for part of the hospital bill. Once health insurance, for which I am extremely grateful, and other discounts I didn't understand were applied, my net bill was a still-painful $3,000. The total cost of surgery included separate bills from the anesthesiologist, the surgeon, and the hospital.

Like most Americans, I think I understand my health insurance plan better than I actually do. This is because I nod off reading the second paragraph of my policy's benefits page, which is a stronger sedative than Ambien or most elephant tranquilizers. (Doctors could prescribe reading your policy before bed; it's extremely nonaddictive and cheaper than sleeping pills.)

Before your surgery, call your insurance company and speak to an actual person. This live person can explain your benefits, deductibles, and out-of-pocket limits while verbally checking that you are still awake. The insurance rep can tell you if your surgeon, hospital, and medical tests are covered and how much you will need to pay. You may want to use your health savings account if you have one through work. Health plans often require preauthorization before surgery, which your doctor's staff can address.

In order to reduce medical costs, ask if presurgery tests are required. For example, if you had a normal electrocardiogram (EKG), which is a test that measures the electrical activity of the heart, within thirty days of your surgery, you might not need another one right before your operation. Inquire if less expensive tests can be done. Could an ultrasound replace an expensive MRI? You can also save money if your surgery is done in an outpatient facility rather than in the hospital.

If you don't have insurance and can't pay your hospital bill, many hospitals have financial-assistance counselors who can offer a discounted payment plan or financial aid. For example, the Hospital for Special Surgery states on its financial assistance web page that it provides financial aid for "medically necessary services based on a patient's financial need and includes a sliding scale discount for patients that qualify." Call your hospital's financial counselors to discuss your options.

Another possibility is to use a crowdfunding platform like GoFundMe, where people raise money by asking friends, family, and complete strangers for donations to help pay for medical care. One friend paid for an experimental medical procedure by creating a personalized fund-raising page on GoFundMe. She described her medical issues in detail, included adorable photos of her children hugging her, and posted and tweeted links to her fund-raising page. Friends and family shared these links via e-mail and social media. She raised over $10,000 in a month.

CHAPTER 5

Preparing Your Mind and Body for Surgery

You'll want to be mentally and physically prepared for surgery. Instead of thinking, "I'm not sure I can really go through with this," like I did, try to focus on how your life will be better after your operation. Visualize strolling along a beautiful beach after your successful hip replacement or digging into a plate of low-fat turkey bacon without passing out once your painful gallbladder is removed.

Mental preparation can be as important as physical preparation. The following section addresses both.

COPING WITH COMMON WORRIES ABOUT ANESTHESIA, PAIN, SCARS, NEEDLES, AND THE KIDS' REACTIONS

ANXIETY ABOUT SURGERY

It's completely normal to have anxiety about an upcoming surgery. You can talk to your doctor or nurse about your concerns. **Breaking down your general fear into a specific fear that can**

be addressed could make you feel better. For example, if you are worried about nausea from the anesthesia, you can talk to your anesthesiologist about getting an antinausea scopolamine patch. If you are worried about pain, ask your medical team to promise to give you the good pain drugs. Your doctor could also prescribe an effective antianxiety medicine that you can take before surgery.

I tried to ignore my surgery anxiety by staying busy. I made eighteen to-do lists prior to my operation. While I didn't complete one-fourth of the tasks, writing the lists, misplacing them, searching the house and car for them, and then recreating the lists kept me occupied. In addition, I scheduled "worry time" on Tuesday nights from 9:30 to 9:45. If I caught myself fretting about my operation on a Sunday morning, I told myself in a stern voice, "Save it for worry time, pal!" After five minutes of Tuesday-night worry time, I ran out of worries and started recycling them, which got repetitive, and I bored myself to sleep. If I woke up anxious in the middle of the night, I tried to use imagery to calm down. I imagined stuffing my worries into a heavy metal box, locking the box, wrapping it in chains, and tossing it off a sailboat into the middle of the ocean. While I sailed away to a sunny island, my worry box sunk to the ocean floor, where it was buried by sand, kelp, and sea boulders.

Distraction can be a tool to cope with presurgery anxiety. Today's ADD-inducing technology can help you get lost in YouTube, Facebook, and the black hole that is Pinterest. Many people find prayer helpful. They give their worries to a higher power. You could also look into meditations on YouTube. Instead of worrying about rolling into the operation room on a gurney, you can try visualizing sandboarding down a soft desert dune or floating down a lazy river on a cushy inner tube.

Anesthesia

General anesthesia is a combination of intravenous drugs and inhaled gasses that ensure you don't feel any pain and are completely unaware of your operation. It is one of the miracles of modern medicine. Before anesthesia was first used in 1846, people chomped on sticks and guzzled whiskey to get through the pain of an operation. Not only were they awake during surgery, but they also had to contend with a massive hangover and extracting wood chips from their gums.

With general anesthesia, once they put a mask on me, I was out in fifty seconds, falling into a deep, dreamless sleep. And when I woke up, which felt like a few seconds later, my three-and-half-hour surgery was over. I felt no pain during surgery and didn't remember a thing.

For some operations, you can opt for an epidural, which is a local spinal anesthetic that numbs the lower half of the body. With an epidural, you can stay awake during your operation. Or you can have twilight anesthesia, also known as conscious sedation, where you don't go deeply unconscious. One of the benefits of twilight anesthesia and epidurals is that you are less likely to have to deal with "anesthesia brain," where you feel groggy after a procedure.

Anesthesiologists and anesthesiologist nurses are extremely well trained, and the nurse stands next to you throughout surgery, monitoring your vital signs and adjusting the drugs so you stay safe and asleep. They can give you a drug sometimes called "happy juice," which made me feel like I had chugged three margaritas. Happy juice is the sedative Versed, and I received it via IV in the preoperating room. It allowed me to relax, open up, and say things to my surgeon such as "your freckle is very beautiful." Fortunately, the operating room, thanks to HIPAA privacy laws, is like Gamblers Anonymous or Las Vegas. Whatever you say there should stay there.

ANESTHESIA BRAIN

Some people get "anesthesia brain" after a major operation with general anesthesia. Anesthesia brain is when you feel woozy, light-headed, and forgetful after surgery. The anesthesia drugs and inhaled gasses that make you unconscious and unable to feel pain can stay in your system. Anesthesia brain can clear within several hours or, in my particular case, last five to seven days. During my bout of anesthesia brain, I had the attention span of a distracted gnat. I did things like leave my cell phone in the vegetable drawer of the fridge and puzzle over the plot of a *Powerpuff Girls* episode. What helped me get over it was resting, drinking lots of water, and letting time pass.

PAIN

The pain medicines you will be given are strong and effective. The medical profession takes pain control very seriously, and many patients, including me, find that postsurgery pain is less significant than what they expected. Each pain-relief drug works differently, and there is a wide variety of medications that can be used to help manage your pain. If one is not working for you, tell your medical team. They could offer a different type of pain medication or possibly change the dose.

The postoperative nurses want you moving and walking around. They are going to get your pain under control so that you can get up and take a stroll. You will hear that you need to "stay ahead of the pain." That means taking your pain medication on schedule. Don't wait until you feel like you have been mauled by a mountain lion to ask for pain control. Pain, like the news of an unchaperoned high school party, can be more difficult to control once it spreads. You will be able to rest better and heal faster when your pain is well managed. If you are very concerned about postsurgery pain, call your doctor or nurse. They can explain the arsenal of pain medications available to help you.

Scars

I am at the skirted-bathing-suit-and-rash-guard-top stage of life. And my eyesight is mediocre. So I rarely have a clear view of my scars. When I do see them, I try to accept them as "tattoos with a story line." If strangers catch a glimpse of my scars, they may think that I'm a woman with an interesting past. Scars can be intriguing and sexy (see model Padma Lakshmi's arm and Harrison Ford's chin). Ultimately, my scars are the result of operations that saved my life. I wouldn't be here today if I didn't have them.

If you end up feeling self-conscious about your scars, keep in mind that they will fade with time, and you may get used to them. There are also many options that could minimize their appearance, such as scar serums, light therapy, lasers, vitamin-E gel, injectable fillers, chemical peels, dermabrasion, medical-grade silicone scar sheets, scar kelp gels, and skin grafts. Consult a dermatologist or plastic surgeon for recommendations for your particular scars, and remember to use sunscreen on them.

NEEDLES

If you are frightened of needles, tell the person who is taking your blood or inserting an IV that you have "needle phobia." ("Phobia" makes it sound official.) She may use a smaller "butterfly" needle and send in the most experienced nurse or phlebotomist—The Vein Whisperer—to do the job. Some medical professionals are gifted at inserting needles. The Vein Whisperer can find a perfect vein by touch and has the superior hand-eye coordination of a sardine har- pooner. I have teeny-tiny veins, except for one giant bulgy one in the crook of my right elbow, which is, not to brag, my Vin Diesel vein. I always recommend that hulking vein as the one to stick, as it boasts a 100 percent success rate.

It helps to look away and distract myself when a needle is being inserted. I text with one hand, count backward from two hundred by sevens, or count the shades of color in a picture on the wall. Before having a routine blood draw, try to drink extra water. Hydration plumps up veins and makes the process, which only takes a few min- utes, go smoothly.

When a nurse had trouble getting blood from my son, we gave her a two-stick limit. After two failed attempts, she agreed to bring in a more experienced nurse, who placed a warm pack on his vein and then did a successful, quick draw. If a medical professional can't complete an uncomfortable procedure after two or three attempts, whether it's drawing blood or pressing hard on your stomach with a giant ultrasound wand in search of a gallstone, speak up. Just say, "This isn't working for me." Ask for a more experienced medical professional to complete the procedure.

TELLING THE KIDS ABOUT YOUR SURGERY

How much information you tell your children about your surgery will depend on their ages. What worked for me was telling them the minimal amount of information while being truthful. My kids didn't need to be burdened with the juicy details about how my catheter would be inserted or the risks associated with my surgery. My husband and I told all three kids at the same time; we wanted them to learn about my upcoming surgery from us and not a friend or relative or each other. I tried to act calm and let them know that we would answer any questions they might have. My children wanted to hear about friends who successfully had the same surgery I was having.

They also wanted to know who would be taking care of them while I was out of commission. My mother-in-law, who is much more fun than I am, watched my kids while I was in the hospital. When the kids weren't in school, she kept them busy at the park, the movies, and self-serve frozen yogurt shops, where they consumed fifty-two different candy toppings with their tablespoon of yogurt. Your recovery can be an opportunity for the kids to spend time bonding with relatives and friends. For a summer operation, my son went to my in-laws' in Chicago for two weeks, and my girls flew to the Jersey Shore to stay with their cousins for three weeks.

During my recovery, the kids stepped up to take on new responsibilities with the pets, laundry, and dishes. Finally, if you have teens, remind them *not* to use Dr. Google on their cell phones. If they want more information about your surgery, they should go to *you*.

TAKING TIME OFF FROM WORK

When you tell your boss that you need time off from work for surgery, it's up to you to decide how much information you want to reveal. You can simply say, "I need six weeks off for major surgery," or get into the specifics of your upcoming operation. Before you tell your supervisor, draft a tentative coverage plan of who could do your work while you are out and how you can adjust work travel if needed. Present this plan right after you ask for your medical leave of absence.

If you have a human resources (HR) department, check with them to determine if you are covered by disability insurance and FMLA (the Family and Medical Leave Act, which allows eligible employees to take unpaid, job-protected leave for specific medical reasons). There may be forms to complete to get coverage. You will need to make sure that all paperwork is signed by your physician and HR has received it. Also, ask HR if you can use sick days and vacation days to cover your time off or if it should be taken as unpaid leave. If you have supplemental disability insurance, it may cover a long recovery period.

GETTING IN SHAPE BEFORE SURGERY

The Mayo Clinic advises that people who eat well, get conditions like diabetes under control, and exercise regularly before surgery recover faster.[1] Some surgeons ask their patients to walk briskly two miles a day for thirty days before surgery. If you are already doing this, great! If your current exercise regimen consists of warming the couch while popping open the cheese puffs, start walking for five minutes at a time and add more each week until you reach a two-mile stroll. Right after surgery, the nurses are going to "strongly encourage" (force) you out of bed and "suggest" (make) you walk, because walking helps circulation, prevents blood clots, and contributes to general healing. It's easier to get out of bed after your operation if you are in decent shape going into surgery.

Your doctor might recommend strength exercises before surgery, which is known as "prehabilitation." For example, if you are having your knees replaced, your doctor might suggest arm-strengthening exercises so you can easily use your crutches after your operation. In addition, some orthopedic surgeons will prescribe a preoperative home visit by a physical therapist. The physical therapist can show patients pre- and postoperative exercises as well as how to correctly use a walker or crutches. You can take the walker and crutches out for a test drive to see if they are the right height and comfortable to use.

STOPPING SMOKING

Doctors recommend that patients stop smoking weeks before surgery. (Check with your surgeon for her specific recommendation.) Smoking can slow wound healing and increase the risk of infection following an operation. Some plastic surgeons refuse to even operate on smokers. And hospitals don't allow smoking. After an operation, who wants to drag an IV pole out to the sidewalk and huddle with other smoking and contagious patients while your hospital gown flaps in the wind? Plus, smoking is ridiculously expensive. Smokers could go on a twenty-one-day cruise to the North Pole or buy a

Korean minicar for what they spend on cigarettes in a year. For information and encouragement on quitting smoking, visit Smokefree.gov or talk to your doctor.

STOPPING MEDICATIONS AND SUPPLEMENTS

Ask your medical team when and if you should stop taking your medications, vitamins, and herbal supplements before your surgery. Doctors usually recommend that patients stop taking blood-thinning medications and all supplements a week or two before an operation. Things like aspirin, fish oil, ibuprofen, and garlic supplements can thin your blood. During surgery, you don't want your blood to be too thin, causing you to bleed excessively, or too thick, causing it to clot too easily. You also don't want to take anything that could interfere with the anesthesia, so be sure to check with your medical team about when to stop taking medications and supplements.

COMPLETING DENTAL WORK

Many doctors suggest that major dental procedures like getting a tooth pulled or a root canal should be completed weeks before your surgery.[2] When you hear this recommendation, you might think, "But don't I have enough on my plate right now? I'm trying to plan for surgery. The dentist is the last person I want to see!" As the owner of sensitive teeth and exposed roots, I also felt this way. (My dentist, in turn, reciprocates these feelings. I make horrible wincing noises as soon as he touches a tooth, and 99.8 percent of my dental work is now delegated to his hygienist, while he hides behind an x-ray machine on the far side of the office.)

But even if my dentist and I dreaded seeing each other, it was important that I completed any major dental work before surgery. My medical team also mentioned that some surgery patients shouldn't have their teeth cleaned or do any kind of dental procedures until two to three months after surgery. That's because bacteria could enter the bloodstream during a dental cleaning and cause an infection. Check with your doctor for her specific recommendations about visiting the dentist.

PREPARING FOR SURGERY IF YOU HAVE A CHRONIC HEALTH CONDITION

If you have a chronic health condition like diabetes, multiple sclerosis, rheumatoid arthritis, or heart issues, make sure that your surgical team is aware of your condition. Broadcast your chronic condition to the nurses, doctors, physical therapists, and everyone you meet in the hospital. This includes your anesthesiologist, who can take precautions during your operation. For example, if you have diabetes, the anesthesiologist can give you insulin during surgery to help control your blood sugar.

In addition, check in with your chronic-condition doctor. She should know about your upcoming surgery. Ask if you need to stop taking medications like blood thinners or other prescription drugs and when you should restart them. For autoimmune diseases like rheumatoid arthritis or lupus, the surgeon and rheumatologist might want to schedule your operation between monthly doses and injections of medications.

WHAT IF I HAVE SLEEP APNEA?

Does your partner complain about your high-decibel snoring accompanied by pauses and snorts? If the answer is yes, talk to your doctors to see if you might have sleep apnea. Sleep apnea is a disorder where you repeatedly stop and start breathing while sleeping. Obstructive sleep apnea is associated with higher postsurgery complications. And it is fairly common. The Mayo Clinic reports that up to one in five older surgical patients have it.[3]

Check with your doctor about your snoring. She might send you to a sleep specialist, who can offer a variety of solutions. If you do have sleep apnea, your anesthesiologist and nurses will take extra measures to make sure your surgery and recovery go smoothly. They might also ask you to bring your CPAP (continuous positive airway pressure) machine with you to the hospital.

How to Really Rest at Home

After major surgery, doctors will recommend that you get plenty of rest for several weeks. But what does "resting" really mean?

Resting is lying down with your feet up while reading, napping, watching TV, listening to music, or doing some other quiet activity. When you are resting, you're not hosting visitors or doing light chores like folding clothes. You might feel well enough to do these things, but that's not considered resting.

After you rest for an hour or so, it's a good idea to get up and walk for a few minutes. While resting is important, short walks improve your circulation and prevent blood clots and pneumonia. You can rest for an hour and then do a lap around the living room before sitting down at the dinner table, or do a little stroll before moving to the couch to watch TV.

If you currently are Superman or Superwoman, successfully juggling a job, family, volunteer commitments, household chores, an exercise program, and an active social life, be prepared to hang up your cape for your recovery. After surgery, you will need to follow your doctor's instructions and take it easy. I picked two things to focus on during my six-week recoveries, my health and my family. My part-time job, volunteer projects, social commitments, and yard work were shelved. I was MIA from the PTA. Moms Night Out became Mom's Night In. Part of my lawn grew into a prairie where little ground squirrels took up residence. Neighbors, colleagues, and friends understood, adjusted, and offered to help. Accept the help; it will make everyone happier.

What to Wear and Not Wear after Surgery

After an operation, doctors recommend that patients wear loose, comfortable clothing that doesn't rub and irritate incisions. Plus, you need room for bandages or a cast. And you want to be able to easily pull your clothes on and off throughout your recovery. For me, that meant donning loose-fitting PJs, oversized nightgowns, roomy sweatshirts, and large granny panties. (No super-slim jeans, jeggings, girdles, or thongs! Repeat to yourself, "Baggy is better!") Like many fashionistas, I layered my silhouette: my large zip-up sweat jacket covered a sack-like nightgown, which lay over my puffy underwear. The good news for those of us with stomach incisions is that granny underwear is back in style. (See the *New York Times* article "Young Women Say No to Thongs!") And it's easy to see why. Comfortable, available in affordable six-packs, and wide enough to reach the seams of your oversized sweat pants, thereby eliminating panty lines, granny panties make sense. I bought mine at Target, where I also purchased four dark-colored, oversized nightgowns. A cross between a tent dress and a muumuu, the nightgowns served as my nightwear, daywear, and napwear.

Men should also wear comfortable recovery clothing, like loose-fitting pants, relaxed-waist sweats, roomy pajamas, stretched-out T-shirts, and oversized button-up shirts. In general, avoid clothing that could put pressure on your stitches or cut off your circulation. Your recovery undergarments will depend on your type of surgery. For heart surgery, boxers that are easy to get on and off are recommended. Loose elastic waistbands are encouraged, and seasoned underwear may be the most comfortable. (Your favorite fraying boxers that should have been tossed out six months ago are perfect.) But for prostate surgery or a vasectomy, snug, supportive briefs that hold up pads or a bag of frozen peas are best.

You might now be thinking, "Enough about underwear. What about shoes, the anchor of all outfits? What should I wear on my feet to accompany my loose longline outer garments?" Keep in mind that fashion rules are meant to be broken. While your recovery clothing embraces the oversized anti-fit style, your shoes do not. You may be unable to bend over to tie your shoelaces for weeks after your operation. Slip-on sneakers or other sturdy flat shoes that fit well are a good choice. Avoid heels, high wedges, and platform shoes until you are off your pain medicines.

Getting a Handicapped Parking Placard

If you are having surgery that will affect your mobility for several weeks, you might want to get a temporary handicapped parking placard. In many states, you can get a handicapped placard from the

Department of Motor Vehicles (DMV). In order to have minimal physical contact with the DMV and avoid waiting in an endless line only to discover that you don't have a necessary form, see if you can get the application for a placard from the DMV's website. Once you complete the form, ask your doctor to sign it. Then determine if you can mail or e-mail the form to your local DMV and if they can mail out your placard.

My mom got a handicapped placard after her knee replacement. She didn't use it all the time, but it helped at crowded malls during the holidays. Instead of searching for her car by clicking the lock button on her key fob and following the piercing chirps and startled shoppers, she could silently and easily locate her vehicle in the well-marked handicapped row. She also used the automatic entrance doors and handicapped restrooms, which have grab bars and higher seats and are usually cleaner than the regular stalls. If you are recovering from major surgery, handicapped access makes life easier.

You will also want to make your recovery at home smooth and unproblematic. You can start this process by reviewing the suggestions in the following section.

CHAPTER 6

Preparing Your Home
for Your Recovery

BEFORE GOING IN FOR SURGERY, set up your recovery home base so that you will have easy access to everything you need. You can do this by cleaning, organizing, and stocking up on household provisions.

While most people recover in their own homes, sometimes it's more convenient to spend the first week recuperating at a relative's house or a friend's apartment. If your main caretaker has small children or other dependents, it might make sense to stay with that person.

CLEANING AND CLEARING

I "clean" my house by stacking magazines, laundry, and toys in distinct piles. Sometimes these piles rest in baskets, and sometimes they stand as little hills of clutter. Before surgery, I whittled away at the hills and applied the principles of a centuries-old Chinese interior design system known as "floor feng shui." This translated into removing the fleet of Barbie Glam Convertibles and residences from the family-room carpet and stuffing them into the hall closet. The last thing I needed after surviving surgery was to trip and impale myself on a Barbie Dreamhouse. I also pulled up electric cords and throw rugs and stacked magazines in the garage so I could easily walk around the first floor of my house. I vacuumed, did laundry, and cleared the stairs. As I shambled around the house during my recovery, I was grateful for the uncluttered floors.

Picking Your Recovery Room

For the first week post–major surgery, you probably won't want to use the stairs more than once a day. (And if you have joint-replacement surgery, you will only want to use stairs that have banisters and are completely clear of clutter.) Ideally, your recovery room will be on the same floor as a bathroom and the kitchen. If your bedroom is on a different floor from the kitchen, you can move a cooler or a minifridge into the bedroom. That way you don't have to hike up and down the stairs every time you want a snack. Also, think about downloading a free walkie-talkie app on your smartphone so you and your helper can have quick communication if he or she resides on a different floor. Another possibility would be to place a rollaway bed or recliner in the family room if it's on the same floor as your kitchen and bathroom.

Stocking Your Recovery Room

The base of your recovery room will be the bed or recliner in which you will rest and sleep. Next to the bed, you'll need an arm's-height table for the TV remote, cell phone, iPad, reading material, water bottle, medications, and whatever else you need frequently during the day and night. You could use a basket to keep everything together and make sure it is within easy reach. You will probably want to have the following items nearby: a TV with a working remote, a good reading lamp, and a laptop to keep you entertained. If you don't have these things, you could look into borrowing them from family members or friends. Keep a small pile of pillows and a wedge on the bed or near the recliner to prop yourself into comfortable positions.

Organizing the Bedroom, Kitchen, Bathroom, and Laundry Area

You'll want to reposition regularly used items throughout your house so that they are within easy reach. Since I couldn't bend down, reach up, or lift anything heavier than a gallon of milk after major surgery, I moved necessities to countertops and waist-high tables. While my feng shui-ed floors were clear, my countertops and tables were covered with plates, clothes, and books, and my house looked like a busy thrift store. (This was "cozy clutter chic," an extreme lived-in look for the home.)

I went through my house room by room and made the following adjustments:

Bedroom: This was my main recovery room. It's on the first floor near the bathroom and kitchen. I set it up like a college dorm room so that I could reach the remote, the phone, food, and drinks without ever leaving my bed. I moved a side table from the living room next to my bed for daily necessities. On top of my dresser, I laid out nightgowns, underwear, socks, and sweatshirts to get me through the first five days of recovery. That way I wouldn't have to lean down and open drawers or rummage through my crowded closet. I also made a trip to the library to borrow books and DVDs. I set these on top of my dresser.

Bathroom: Put toiletries that you regularly use on the bathroom counter. I bought facial wipes since I couldn't lean over the sink to wash my face. If your doctor says that you cannot shower for a while after your surgery, you might want to purchase dry shampoo and baby wipes. I laundered enough towels and linens for the first week of my recovery and made sure they were easy to reach. Some patients stick a plastic lawn chair or plastic stool in the shower in case they feel light-headed under the hot water and want to sit down. Your doctor might also recommend a nonslip mat and safety grab bars for the shower. (You can find grab bars for about twenty dollars at Home Depot.) Finally, depending on your type of surgery, some doctors recommend a raised toilet seat with arms so you don't strain your back, knees, and abdominal muscles.

Kitchen: It's a good idea to clean out the fridge and freezer before your surgery. You don't want anything in there that could make you sick during your recovery. Toss out food that is past its expiration date, leftovers from last season's Super Bowl party, and anything sprouting green stubble. I purchased two fifteen-dollar OXO Good Grips spinning lazy Susans for my refrigerator shelf so I wouldn't have to reach far into the refrigerator. I placed cold snacks like yogurts and protein drinks on the lazy Susans. I set granola bars and other snacks on the counters and pulled out plastic plates and cups, which are lighter than china. Finally, you might want to pull the coffee maker, toaster, and microwave forward so you can easily reach them.

Laundry area: I did as much laundry as possible before going to the hospital. I also stocked up on detergent so my school-aged kids could do the laundry while I was out of commission. Since their experience with the laundry process was digging out "good jeans" and pieces of sports uniforms from the dryer, I gave them basic laundry lessons. I explained that all clothing emitting strong fumes must be washed in hot water. (This was a revelation! As was the existence of the dryer's lint screen.) We reviewed that wet laundry left in the washing machine for days will mildew and that damp clothes should *not* be stuffed into drawers. This last issue surfaced when we ran a practice load, which I recommend doing. It's also helpful to stick reminder Post-its on the washer and dryer. My children did a good job with the laundry, which can be a complex process potentially fraught with errors.

Once your house is set up, try using your crutches or walker while completing everyday chores. (If you're getting shoulder surgery, use your unaffected arm to do daily activities.) Brush your teeth and get in and out of the shower. Go to the kitchen and make a sandwich. Then move items around or modify things as needed to make your postsurgery life easier.

Helpful Grabbers

After my major surgeries, I was forbidden to reach up or lean over, because my internal and external stitches were slowly healing. In order to pick things up that fell on the floor or were too high to reach, I relied on a mechanical device technically called a grabber thingy. Grabbers are about two feet long with a handle you squeeze on one end to activate the clamp on the other end. You can purchase one at Walmart or Target for about twelve dollars.

When something vitally important like *People* magazine slid off the bed and onto the floor, I whipped out my grabber and easily picked it up. I also used my grabber to remove items on high shelves, pull clothes out of the dryer, and put on my sneakers. By the second week of recovery, I was emotionally attached to my grabber and slept with it at the foot of my bed. Like my childhood "blankie," I needed to know where it was at all times. I ended up buying two more grabbers from Amazon. That way, if my first grabber fell to the floor, I wouldn't panic; I could use my second or third one to grab it.

Stocking Up on Easy Meals and Protein Snacks

High-protein snacks are not just for bodybuilders or teenage boys hoping to sprout muscles. The hospital dietician told me that patients need protein after major surgery to speed healing and repair tissue. The best sources of protein are eggs, meat, fish, dairy products, soy, and nuts. (Besides protein, vitamin C and zinc can help with healing. The Cleveland Clinic offers nutrition guidelines to improve wound healing on their website, http://my.clevelandclinic.org/.)

Before stocking up on the suggested items below, check with your medical team to see if you will have any dietary restrictions during your recovery and how much protein they recommend that you get.

Snacks with Protein
* Yogurt
* Protein bars, like crunchy Power Bars
* Granola bars that have protein, like Kind Bars
* Hard-boiled eggs
* Protein drinks or protein powder to mix into drinks
* Peanut butter crackers
* Hummus and chips
* Apples and peanut butter or any kind of nut butter
* High-protein pretzels, like Newman's Own
* Precooked grilled chicken strips, like Applegate Farms

- Cottage cheese with fruit
- Cans or bags of mixed nuts
- Prepared or canned chili
- Frozen breakfast sandwiches with eggs and meat
- Frozen edamame (soybeans)
- Turkey jerky
- Rotisserie chicken you can slice when hungry
- Turkey, ham, and chicken salad sandwiches

Most of the meals below can be frozen ahead of your surgery. You can make them from scratch or find them at your local supermarket or Trader Joe's. Pop them into the microwave for a quick lunch or dinner.

Easy Meals with Protein

- Cheese or meat tortellini that you can microwave
- Meat lasagna, like Stouffer's
- Chicken or beef enchiladas
- Chicken or beef taquitos
- Turkey or beef chili
- Meatballs
- High-protein pasta
- Precooked chicken and turkey sausages, like Aidell's or Applegate Farms
- Frozen quiche
- Chicken pot pie
- Meatloaf
- Trader Joe's Mandarin Orange Chicken
- Trader Joe's Tarte d'Alsace (ham, gruyere cheese, and caramelized onion pizza—I like to top it with a fried egg)
- Sandwiches—fillings like turkey, ham, or chicken, or egg salad, chicken salad, or tuna salad

SMOOTH MOVES

Your bowels slow down during surgery, and many pain drugs are constipating. This may come as an indelicate surprise, but some people do not poop for five or more days after an operation. It can be uncomfortable to be "stuck in neutral," as one nurse put it. **Fiber is your friend** postsurgery and can get things moving. (Also, drinking a lot of water, walking, and taking Miralax can help.)

After reviewing the recommended high-fiber foods listed below, you might wrinkle your nose and wonder why, with all the gene-splicing, GMO-creating food technology available today, have they not figured out how to make high-fiber foods taste like jelly donuts? They are working on this! In the meantime, many high-fiber foods taste better. According to Consumer Reports, fiber cereals have improved dramatically from the past, when they used to taste more like straw than grain.[1] Now many are officially rated "very good."

High-Fiber Foods
High-fiber cereal, such as Raisin Bran, All-Bran, or oatmeal
Prunes
High-fiber bread or waffles, such as Thomas' High Fiber
    English Muffins, Ezekiel Breads, or Kashi waffles
Raisins
Craisins (dried cranberries)
Kiwis
Smooth Move tea
Bran muffins
Pear or prune juice
Coffee

Grapes and grape juice
High-fiber granola bars

Lining Up Medical Equipment

Ask your nurse what type of medical equipment you will need and if you should bring it to the hospital. A walker or crutches might be covered by your insurance company. Often a nurse can line these up for you. If not, see if you can borrow them from friends and family. You can also rent medical equipment like a scooter or a knee walker online at a reasonable price. Or check to see if a local Goodwill or Red Cross offers gently used, "preloved" crutches and walkers. Another possibility would be to search a neighborhood website like Nextdoor.com for medical equipment. Once you have your equipment, try it out to see if any adjustments need to be made.

Some people who have shoulder, stomach, or breast surgery feel more comfortable sleeping in a recliner. And they find it easier to slide out of a recliner than a bed. For abdominal or heart surgery, the doctors will usually want you to sleep on your back, and wedge pillows might make you feel more comfortable. Check with your nurse to see if she has postsurgery sleeping tips, and then, if needed, look into borrowing a recliner or extra pillows.

What to Do When Lying Around Recovering

Recovering from surgery gives you the gift of "me time." You will have the opportunity to slow down, take a break from your hectic schedule, and focus on yourself and your needs. Granted, you may be uncomfortable and exhausted during your me time, but at least you'll finally get some. Think about what you'll want to do while sprawled on the couch. How about catching up on Netflix shows and movies, exploring new hobbies, and calling old friends?

During my recovery me time, I watched comedies, read magazines, contacted friends, and ignored social media. (Who wants to see evidence of the parties you're missing or another photo of someone else's sandy feet on a lounge chair on a Mexican beach?) I tried to create a positive recovery bubble for myself. That meant doing things I enjoyed and avoiding depressing movies, Morrissey, and phone calls from telemarketers trying to loan me money.

The following is a list of activities I thought about doing while reclining with my feet up, (I actually did four of them.) Do many, do one, or do none. There is no pressure, no worries—it's your time.

* Read magazines and books.
* Watch TV shows and movies.
* Shop in bed.
* Listen to audiobooks, music, and podcasts.
* Explore Pinterest.
* Call and text old friends.
* Learn, via YouTube or an MIT Online honors course, how to use the four remotes required to turn on my television. Stop relying on my eleven-year-old to magically juggle the remotes so I can watch *The Bachelor* and his sister can shimmy to Dance Dance Revolution.
* Play Sudoku or solitaire or complete crossword puzzles.
* Do craft projects or make beaded gifts. When our loved ones say that they are thrilled to receive crafty homemade presents, they usually are just being polite. (They really wanted a

Cheesecake Factory gift card.) An exception to this is in the senior community, where "brag-bead" necklaces handcrafted by grandchildren are the ultimate status symbol. (The bigger and brighter the beads, the better they can be seen over trifocals.) Each brag-bead necklace enables the wearer to tell friends, cashiers, and anyone who comes within a hundred yards all about her grandchild's jewelry-design skills, bead-stringing giftedness, and future as Tiffany's CEO. My mom coveted one for years, and now I would finally have time to help my kids make one for her.

* Organize seventeen years' worth of printed and digital photos.
* Meditate.
* Take an online class. Lie on the couch, log on to Babble.com from my laptop, and learn basic Spanish. (I did not do this. I had anesthesia brain and spent my time googling, in my native English, *US* magazine vocabulary words such as "bae" and "twerking.")
* Play video games.
* Learn free-form embroidery or knitting via YouTube.
* Plan and research a vacation.
* Hang out and enjoy my creative kids. Draw, read, watch a movie or cartoon together, view their beatboxing and moonwalking contests.

CHAPTER 7

Preparing for Your Hospital Stay

YOUR SURGICAL NURSE SHOULD GIVE you information about how
to prepare for your hospital stay and recovery. She should tell you
things like how long you will be in the hospital and whether you
will need a special diet during your recovery. Some hospitals offer
surgery preparation classes, and others, like UCLA Health, have informational videos on their websites. Each doctor will have her own
instructions, and you should follow what your medical team recommends for your operation.

The following is an overview of what I experienced and learned
as a patient and as an advocate for my son during his elbow surgery.
The order and timing of events might be different or not applicable
to your specific situation. While everyone's hospital experience will
be unique, it's helpful to have a general idea of what to expect.

WHAT HAPPENS AT A PREADMISSION APPOINTMENT?

Three days before my surgery, I had a preadmission appointment
at the hospital. I brought my insurance card, credit cards, ID, and
a list of every medication and supplement I took. The first part of
the appointment was with the financial counselor. She inputted my

personal and insurance information into her computer and presented my huge hospital bill with a Vulcan-like calmness that comes from delivering bad news eight hours a day, 340 days a year.

After recovering from my meeting with the financial counselor, I saw the preadmitting nurse. She reviewed my health history, my medications, my allergies, and the details of my upcoming operation. She then took my vitals, a urine sample, and two vials of blood, and determined whether I needed a quick chest x-ray or other tests before my surgery. Basically, she was checking for anything that could affect the success of my upcoming operation and getting my baseline health information. This was the time for me to reveal all of my health issues, however trivial or embarrassing, as well as report any supplements I had recently ingested. It was my job to keep my team informed about my current health, medical history, supplements, and allergies. I also needed to confess whether I skipped doses of my medications or started any new habits that could affect my health.

The nurse concluded the appointment by handing me a bottle of pink Hibiclens antibacterial soap to wash with on the morning of my operation. She also gave me a page of written instructions and reminded me not to drink or eat anything after midnight before my operation.

Donating Blood to Yourself

Some medical professionals suggest that patients consider donating their own blood to themselves ahead of surgery. This is called an autologous donation, and it can be nice to have on hand in case it is needed. (I did not donate my own blood prior to my surgeries. I was anemic and did not want my weak, recycled blood back.) If you are interested in an autologous donation, talk to your doctor. The American Red Cross website, redcross.org, has information on donating blood to yourself. You can donate blood weeks before your surgery as long as you meet certain guidelines and have a doctor's prescription.

Do You Want a Hospital Roommate?

Hospitals usually have private or semiprivate rooms. The semiprivate rooms are for two people. They have two beds separated by a thin curtain. Everyone—nurses, doctors, and visitors—likes to pretend that the curtain is a wall and that your semiprivate room is really a private room. They hang signs on your curtain reminding people to wash their hands before entering this "room." Well-educated medical professionals will act like your curtain is a soundproof structure with a door and say "Knock, knock" before entering. But at some point you will realize, "Aha! They are just kidding! My curtain is a flimsy piece of fabric that allows me to hear my roommate's sensitive physical exams and late-night phone calls to her boyfriend."

When I'm feeling ill, I prefer to be alone, mute, and motionless in a dark room. So I requested a private room when I scheduled my surgeries. The advantages of having a private room are that you sleep better (relatively) and you don't have to chat with your roommate's relatives or share a bathroom. If you want a private room, make sure to ask for one when you schedule surgery and confirm it when you check in upon admission. Also, check to see if your insurance will cover a private room. Sometimes you have to pay extra, such as forty dollars per day. The additional cost could be well worth the privacy.

Usually, single-occupancy rooms are filled first, and then the semiprivates are filled. There is a possibility that you could win the lottery of hospital room assignments and get a semiprivate room but never have a roommate. Or you might have a roommate for only one night. If you do get a semiprivate room, try to grab the bed by the window so you have a view and a tad more privacy. If you have trouble sleeping with a roommate, let the nurse manager know. Ask her to move you to a private room as soon as one becomes available.

After her knee-replacement surgeries, my mom, who is an incredibly resilient patient, had several roommates at her rehabilitation center. There were social upsides of sharing a room. Mom and her roommate could discuss the merits of the cafeteria's cream of celery soup and jointly complain about the room's temperature. Since my mom doesn't like to be alone, she was comforted that her roommate could call the nurse if she had an unexpected complication or rolled out of bed. And my mom experienced "comparison compassion." Some of her roommates were recovering from serious conditions like strokes. After hearing their health woes, her double knee-replacement surgery didn't seem so bad.

PACKING-FOR-THE-HOSPITAL CHECKLISTS
I wore comfortable, loose sweats, a baggy T-shirt, a large zip-up sweat jacket, warm socks, and slip-on sneakers to the hospital. I also wore my glasses, since you can't wear contacts in surgery. The following are lists of items I packed.

I carried these items in my purse:

* Insurance card
* Driver's license

- Small amount of cash (around twenty dollars)
- Credit card
- Cell phone with headphones (you might want to download an app of soothing sounds)
- Lip balm
- Directions to the hospital
- A terrifying murder mystery to keep my mind occupied in the presurgery waiting room

I had these items in a small overnight bag:

- Loose nightgown
- Granny panties and socks
- Earplugs
- Eye mask for sleeping
- Cell phone charger
- Toothbrush and toothpaste
- Disinfectant wipes with bleach to wipe down everything in my hospital room
- Big bottle of hand sanitizer
- Lifestyle magazines with large pictures and short captions for postsurgery anesthesia brain

☐ Check with your surgeon on whether you should bring any medications that you are currently taking that she has approved.
☐ Bring your living will or advance directive if you have one.
☐ Bring this book.
☐ If you use a CPAP machine for sleep apnea, you might need to bring it to the hospital. Check with your surgeon's nurse about this.

Do **not** bring valuables to the hospital such as jewelry, lots of cash, watches, hair pieces, or credit cards.

I left a small travel pillow in my car to wedge between the seat belt and my stitches during the ride home:

Here are some things my hospital provided:

* Revealing hospital gowns
* Nonslip socks
* Small bottles of shampoo
* Small toothbrush and toothpaste
* Soap
* Antiseptic gel nailed to the wall
* Disposable mesh underwear—these were comfortable and could be sexy under different circumstances

Day-and-Night-before-Surgery Checklist

The following checklist is based on my doctor's instructions for what I needed to do the day and night before surgery. Check with your surgeon's nurse for your specific instructions.

☐ **Do not eat or drink anything (including your regular medicine, water, gum, mints, or hard candy) after midnight the day of surgery, unless you are directed otherwise**.

☐ Charge your cell phone.

☐ Check that your bag is packed.

☐ Make sure you know how to get to the hospital (and give yourself plenty of time to get there).

Morning-of-Surgery Checklist

☐ Take a shower the morning of surgery, because this could help minimize the chance of infection. My doctor had me wash with Hibiclens, an antibacterial soap. With my surgeon's permission, I took a heartburn pill with two sips of water. I brushed my teeth but did my best not to swallow water.

☐ Go au naturel. Do not put on makeup, nail polish, acrylics, jewelry, wigs, fake eyelashes, barrettes, or contacts. No hair extensions or toupees. Remove piercings. Health-care providers don't want anything to fall into your incision or serve as a conduit for germs. Your nails should be polish-free because they will check your circulation via your nailbeds. Small particles of makeup could get into your eyes and irritate them when you don't have a blink reflex while under anesthesia. A giant pair of sunglasses and a baseball cap can serve as your makeup and hairstyle.

☐ Leave valuables (watches and jewelry) at home.

☐ Check that you have your ID, insurance card, cell phone, phone charger, packed overnight bag, books and magazines, and a small amount of cash.

☐ Dress in loose, comfortable clothing and slip-on shoes.

What to Do If You Get Sick before Surgery

What if you get a fever or a stomach bug the night before or the morning of your surgery? Call your surgeon's office right away and let them know about your illness. Your doctor may want to delay your operation. But don't assume that your surgery will be postponed. If the operation is medically urgent, she may want to go ahead with it.

How to Reduce the Chance of a Medical Error

One of the best ways to reduce the chance of a medical error is to speak up when you have a question or something doesn't seem right. Remind your hospital advocate it's also her job to speak up and communicate your health information, such as allergies or drug reactions. Ask your nurse about the pills she gives you—what's in them and what they do. If your doctor hasn't reviewed the results of an important blood test, follow up with her.

The following medical error reduction tips are based on recommendations from the Agency for Healthcare Research and Quality.[1]

Medical Error Reduction Tips:

- Before surgery, make sure that all of your doctors know about any prescription and over-the-counter medicines and dietary supplements you take, such as vitamins and herbs.
- Make sure that all the health professionals involved in your care know about your allergies and any history of reactions to anesthesia or other drugs. Do not assume that everyone knows everything they need to. For example, make sure your surgeon and anesthesiologist are both aware of your penicillin allergy.
- When your nurse gives you a pill or medicine through an IV, ask her the name of the drug, what it is used for, and how often you need to take it. If you are groggy, your hospital advocate should ask on your behalf.
- Ask for information about your medicines in terms you can understand. Ask about them at the hospital and when you

receive them from your local pharmacist. Your pharmacist is a font of drug information. Take the time to review your prescriptions with her.

♦ You and your surgeon should agree and be clear on exactly what will be done during your operation. The American Academy of Orthopaedic Surgeons urges its members to sign their initials directly on the surgical site. Don't be surprised if your doctor whips out a Sharpie pen and writes on your body in the pre-op room.

♦ Don't chat excessively with doctors or nurses during a procedure. This can be distracting for the medical professionals, who need to concentrate.

♦ If you have a test, ask for the results. No news isn't necessarily good news.

♦ Know that more is not always better. Find out why a test, treatment, or medicine is needed and how it can help you.

♦ Spend as little time in the hospital as possible. Ask if your medical tests and procedures can be done on an outpatient basis.

♦ If you don't see your medical team washing their hands before they touch you, speak up. See the section below for tips on how to do this.

How to Avoid a Hospital-Acquired Infection

Hospitals are convention centers for germs. (There are superbugs in hospitals that we really don't want to know about and are better left to the infectious-disease professionals in white hazmat suits.) Hospitals do their best to reduce infections by enforcing strict handwashing policies, administering antibiotics in IVs during surgery, and isolating contagious patients. **But the sooner you**

can get safely discharged to your comparatively low-germ home, the better. (Insurance companies love this advice.) Also, if your surgery is delayed for a day, ask if you can go home. If you have to stay in the hospital, request to have your operation as soon as possible.

Because I desperately wanted to avoid a hospital-acquired infection, I took the following steps, which were based on my nurses' recommendations and the nonprofit Committee to Reduce Infectious Deaths, which offers tips on its website, http://hospitalinfection.org/protect/patients.

Steps to Avoid a Hospital-Acquired Infection:

* On my surgeon's recommendation, I washed and showered with Hibiclens, a soap that can help prevent infections, the morning of surgery.
* I did not shave for four days before surgery per my surgeon's recommendation. Micro nicks or cuts can be conduits for infection.
* I brought two tubs of antibacterial wipes with bleach to the hospital. I asked my husband to wipe down anything in my hospital room that we would touch, such as the TV remote, call buttons, the menu, bed rails, chair arms, door handles, sink handles, the tray table, etc., as well as our cell phones. I used my elbow to touch elevator buttons.
* I did not touch my IVs or incision. Tell your nurse if your bandage becomes loose or wet.
* I used antibacterial foam or soap and water before every hospital meal and every time I got out of bed. I also bugged my

husband to use the antibacterial foam, which was nailed to the wall. If you have visitors, ask them to wash their hands before they touch you or anything that you touch, like your TV remote or phone.

* Handwashing is essential in reducing hospital-acquired infections. You will see signs all over the hospital that shout, "STOP! DID YOU WASH YOUR HANDS?" Your doctors and nurses should wash their hands before they touch you or change any IV or catheter. My medical team almost always washed or foamed up in front of me. If they didn't, I tried to approach the issue in a tactful, nonconfrontational way. Here are some creative ways to bring up handwashing with your medical team:

  * Squint and say, "Doctor, my eyesight is not great; I'm not sure if I saw you wash your hands. Did you wash them in the hallway?"

  * Mention to the nurses that your hands look younger and suppler since you were admitted to the hospital. Chalk this up to the moisturizer in the antibacterial foam. Show off the back of your hands like Palmolive Madge and declare, "It's the *foam*! It softens hands. You need to try it right now!"

  * Be direct and inquire, "Doctor, would you mind washing your hands in front of me before you examine me?" Then blame your question directly on Dr. Oz. Explain that Dr. Oz is your personal teledoctor, and he told you, through your thirty-six-inch screen, to ask this question. Mention that you follow all of Dr. Oz's advice, not just because he is as handsome as George Clooney, but also because he saved your life when he revealed that your apple juice, sitting innocently in the cupboard, was actually trying to

kill you. (See the "Arsenic in Apple Juice" episode of *The Dr. Oz Show*.)

* I asked that tubes entering my body, like catheters, be taken out as soon as I didn't need them. The risk of infection increases the longer a catheter is in.[2]

* When eating in the hospital, I kept my utensils on my plate. I didn't let them rest on the table or bed or let anyone else use them.

* I took my antibiotics as prescribed and asked my doctor if I could take a probiotic with them.

* I asked if I could avoid taking proton pump inhibitor (PPI) heartburn medicine unless medically necessary. According to the *Journal of General Internal Medicine*, PPIs can increase the risk of pneumonia and *Clostridium difficile* (a type of bacteria) infection after an operation.[3]

* I got out of the hospital as quickly as I safely could.

* Once I was home, I changed out of all the clothes I had worn in the hospital and had them washed twice in hot water. Because I am a paranoid human being, I asked my husband to wipe down our cell phones, laptop, and anything else we brought home from the hospital.

CHAPTER 8

Your Hospital Stay

It's showtime! This section provides an overview of what happens during a hospital stay, and it's based on my experiences. While you will have your own unique hospital experience, I hope the following will give you an idea of what to expect.

Day of Surgery: Checking In at Admissions

I arrived two hours before my surgery to check in at the admissions area. After showing my driver's license and insurance card to the cheery admissions lady, I signed a consent form and an agreement to pay for medical expenses that were not covered by my health insurance. I received an ID bracelet that had my name, date of birth, and ID number, and a colored bracelet indicating a drug allergy. (Check that all the information on your bracelet is correct.)

Throughout this give-and-take, I remained surprisingly composed. Surgery was something I just needed to get through. "Thousands of people have successful surgeries every day," I silently reminded myself. "I have a great doctor. I trust her. I will be absolutely fine."

I continued self-soothing until the admissions lady asked with a sweet smile, "Kaye, do you have a living will?"

Instead of blinking back tears and searching for the nearest exit sign, I should have remembered that hospital policies require that patients be asked if they have advance directives or living wills. These legal documents describe your medical care preferences if you are unable to make decisions for yourself. (For more information, the Mayo Clinic website has a good overview of living wills. They suggest you complete one before checking in to the hospital.) Asking patients about a living will is simply a hospital policy, like requesting that visitors don't smoke or insisting that patients wear ugly nonskid socks. It was not a sign that my operation was going to go off the rails. In fact, my surgery went well.

DAY OF SURGERY: MOVING TO THE PREOPERATIVE WAITING ROOM AND HOLDING AREA

Next, a nurse called my name and escorted me and my husband to a higher floor of the hospital and into a preoperative waiting room, where family members wait during their loved one's surgery. Your advocate will spend 90 percent of his time waiting around. He will wait while you check in, wait while you have your operation, wait while you sleep, wait while you do physical therapy, and wait for your discharge papers. Remind him to bring a book, a laptop, a cell phone and charger, and anything else he can think of to keep busy. Do not rely on the hospital's magazine supply for entertainment. All the good magazines have been "permanently borrowed" by fellow patients. What remains in the waiting rooms are tattered issues of *WebMD* and pamphlets on managing stress printed during the first Bush administration.

A nurse called my name and took me into the preoperative hold-ing area, which had three other patients in curtained-off spaces pre-paring for surgery. It was comforting to know that I was not alone. Roughly forty-nine million inpatient surgeries are performed in the United States every year, according to the latest data from the National Center for Health Statistics. That breaks down to about fifty-six hundred surgeries per hour. All across America, thousands of people were sharing my presurgery jitters.

The nurse took my blood pressure, temperature, and pulse and asked questions about when I last ate, what medications I was tak-ing, and what my health history was. She also asked my name and birthday, if I was pregnant, and what operation I was having while she looked at the information on my wristband to make sure I was having the right surgery.

The nurse then gave me a hospital gown, nonskid socks, a blue shower cap, and a giant clear ziplock bag. Per her instructions, I took off my clothes, underwear, shoes, and socks and stuffed them into the ziplock bag. Your advocate will carry this bag around with him for the next several hours. People in the waiting room, cafeteria, and wherever else he travels will have a clear view of its contents, so wear good underwear to the hospital.

I put on the nonskid socks, plastic blue shower cap, and hospital gown. The hospital gown is a short, one-piece garment that has the texture and thickness of a Bounty paper towel. Its deceivingly simple sack design, originally conceived of by potato farmers, has been con-fusing patients for decades. Don't worry if your gown's ties are in the front when they should go in the back, or if you stick your legs through the arm holes. The nurses will correct you. The shower cap, which is technically called a "bouffant," keeps your hair out of the surgeon's way during the operation. Doctors don't want hair ending up in your incision and possibly contributing to an infection. While the shade of baby blue and height of the bouffant cap were not particularly flattering, it was comfortable, effective, and flexible, expanding to cover a range of hair heights, from my medium-length locks to the big hair of eighties rock stars.

Once I was in my cap and gown, the pre-op nurse told me to "relax on the gurney." While this sounds like an oxymoron, it was possible when she wrapped me in perfectly warm blankets from the blanket warmer. The blanket warmer looks like a large aluminum Easy-Bake Oven and is the best thing about being in the hospital. It bakes blankets to the temperature of a wonderfully warm shower. (One of the first things I did when I returned home was to search Amazon for a hospital-grade blanket warmer, but they were five thousand dollars above my budget.) I enjoyed baked blankets during my hospital stay, and I learned that keeping warm right before and after surgery can reduce the chance of infection and help your body heal.[1]

Next, the anesthesiologist stopped by and introduced himself. He asked rapid questions about my health, allergies, and previous experience with anesthesia, and quickly explained some of the risks of anesthesia. He also handed me a consent form that I scanned and signed. The anesthesiologist's pager was buzzing throughout this exchange. He would look at his pager, dash away midsentence, return five minutes later, speak a sentence or two, get paged, and run away again. Finally, he disappeared altogether. So I never heard about *all* the risks of anesthesia. But my anesthesiologist was clearly in high demand, which was a good sign. Plus, I was on a rolling gurney, in a hospital gown, wearing a blue bouffant cap. I was ready to go and all in for the anesthesia drugs, no matter what the risks entailed. (This is not ideally what you want to happen. It would be preferable to meet the anesthesiologist a few days ahead of surgery to discuss your concerns and understand all the risks associated with anesthesia.)

An anesthesiology nurse, also known as a certified registered nurse anesthesiologist, calmly introduced himself and told me he was going to start an IV by sticking a small needle into a vein on the top of my left hand. (I averted my eyes to the murder mystery while he did this.) The IV is a plastic tube that delivers solutions to keep you hydrated and pain-free during surgery. Once the IV is in, the nurse tapes it to your hand using an entire jumbo roll of strong white medical tape. This is done so that the IV will stay in during surgery and your entire hospital stay.

The nurse put monitoring equipment—an inflatable blood-pressure cuff, pulse monitor, and heart monitor sticky patches—on me. I was given an antinausea scopolamine patch to wear behind my ear. (This patch is also prescribed for seasickness on cruises. It can cause dry mouth, but it is very effective for nausea.) The anesthesiology nurse reassured me that he would be at my side during the whole operation, monitoring my vital signs. He also answered any last-minute questions that I had.

Then my surgeon came by to say a quick hello and announce that everything was going to go great. My surgeon confirmed the type of operation I was having and drew on me with a felt-tip marker to indicate where incisions should go. (Just as a reminder.)

My husband was brought in for about five minutes to chat and wish me luck. During this time, the anesthesiology nurse put some happy juice (Versed) into my IV. I was wheeled into the operating room, where the nurses and doctors were wearing caps, gowns, booties, eyeglasses, and face masks. They were busy preparing shiny surgical instruments. (And I was busy enjoying the happy juice.) The temperature was cool in the operating room. The nurse anesthesiologist told me he was going to have me count backward. I fell asleep at that point. When I woke up, my three-and-half-hour surgery was over.

After the surgery was done, the surgeon spoke to my husband in a private consultation room to let him know that everything went fine. Your advocate should ask if the operation was successful and if anything unexpected came up that you should know about.

Waking Up in the Recovery Area

The recovery room, also known the postoperative room, can be a private room or a large room with portioned spaces for several patients. It's usually right near the operating room. When I woke up in the recovery room, I felt groggy, as if I had woken up from a long nap. I had deep a sense of relief that the surgery was over and there was little pain, since the anesthesia was still in my system. I wore a blood-pressure cuff and finger pulse monitor, and my IV was delivering medicine and saline. Sequential compression devices were wrapped around my legs to prevent blood clots. Postsurgery recovery time varies from person to person, and it could be an hour or so before your advocate can visit you in the recovery room.

The recovery room nurse checked my vital signs and repeatedly asked, "Kaye, are you awake? How are you feeling, Kaye?" While I heard her questions, I could only respond in short words, as if I were a baby robot learning to speak. I uttered, "Awake," "Done," and "Cold." The nurse understood that I was cold, which is a normal reaction to anesthesia, and wrapped me in warm blankets. If you are in pain, let the nurses know, and they can adjust your pain medicines. My nurse told me to take deep breaths and cough to remove congestion and anesthesia from my lungs. When I hacked like a three-packs-a-day smoker, she congratulated me with, "Good cough! Can you do another?"

Besides an IV, you may have some of the following medical devices attached to you when you wake up from surgery. It will depend on the type of surgery you have and your personal health history. Between my anesthesia and pain drugs, I barely felt them.

Blood-pressure cuff: This was placed on my upper arm and automatically inflated and recorded my blood pressure on a monitor.

Pulse oximeter: A pulse oximeter monitors the saturation of oxygen in your blood. It looks like a fat clothespin and was gently clipped onto my finger.

Urinary (Foley) catheter: A urinary catheter is a thin rubber tube that removes urine (pee) from the bladder while a patient is under anesthesia. Your bladder, like the rest of you, goes to sleep during an operation. The Cleveland Clinic's online Health Dictionary explains, "The catheter tube goes into your urethra and up to your bladder, and is held in place by a small, water-filled balloon." The catheter handles fluid output, which goes into a clear bag, and enables you to rest in bed without having to get up to use the bathroom.

While that sounds well and good, I was not looking forward to having a catheter. The mechanics of it just seemed off. Everything normally flows *out* of your bladder and urethra, often at a high velocity; nothing goes in. And my urethra didn't seem like a particularly roomy organ. How would a tube and a mini water balloon fit through it? While I never understood the technicalities of the catheter, it worked fine. And it turned out to be a complete nonevent. My surgeon put the catheter in while I was under anesthesia, and I did not feel it during surgery or when it was later removed.

Oxygen mask: Oxygen helps clear the anesthesia from your lungs. The mask resembles what you hope and pray will never pop out from your airplane's overhead compartment. I woke up with an oxygen mask over my mouth and nose and kept it on until my vitals were checked. According to the *Journal of the American Medical Association*, oxygen can help reduce post-op infections.[2] The oxygen was odorless and easy to breathe. It was removed about thirty minutes after I woke up.

Heart monitor: Small sticky pads may still be attached to your chest so that your heartbeat can be seen on a monitoring screen. The pads feel like absolutely nothing. I forgot their existence until I found three still stuck to my chest two days after discharge.

Drains: After some surgeries, drains are used to direct fluid away from the incisions. The drains, which are usually inserted under the incision, help speed healing and reduce infection. Drains may be removed before you leave the hospital, or sometimes stay in until you have a follow-up visit with your doctor.

Sequential compression device (SCD): This looks like a long rectangular version of the arm floaties little kids wear in a pool to swim away from their parents into the deep end. The compression device prevents blood clots by wrapping around your legs and inflating and deflating in intervals. This felt like a light massage. (You could shut your eyes and try to imagine that a handsome nurse, a Fabio in scrubs, is rubbing your calves.) My compression leg sleeves were attached with Velcro tabs, and I undid them when I had to take a walk or go to the bathroom. I wore them for my entire hospital stay.

Patient-controlled analgesia (PCA) pump: A PCA pump administers a small amount of morphine or another strong pain medicine directly through the IV into your bloodstream. When I pushed the button on my PCA pump, my pain was reduced in forty seconds. The morphine is premeasured, so I couldn't give myself too much. The advantage of a pump is that the patient controls the pain medicine and doesn't have to wait for a nurse to provide a pain pill or injection. I loved my morphine pump, perhaps a tad too much, so it was probably for the best when it was taken away two days after my operation.

Bandages and dressings: Bandages and dressings are used to cover and protect your incision and promote healing. Many surgeons use stitches, also known as sutures, that dissolve over time and don't have to be removed. Depending on the location and nature of your incisions, your surgeon might use surgical glue, Steri-Strips, or tape to close the surgical wound. You might be asked to leave the bandages and dressing alone, or your doctor might tell you to change them every few days. When you change your dressings, you may see little nylon threads on or near your incision. Do not touch or pull on the little threads to see where they lead. Just leave them alone. They will dissolve, fall off, or be removed during your recovery.

Incentive spirometer: I was also handed an incentive spirometer. I was supposed to take ten breaths with it every one to two hours.

The incentive spirometer encourages you to take long, slow, deep breaths. Deep breaths help clear out mucus and anesthesia from your lungs and prevent pneumonia. The spirometer is a plastic beaker with an attached tube that you hold to your mouth. As you inhale a deep breath, an indicator ball or disc slowly rises, showing the depth of your inhalation. It's like sucking in the air from a helium balloon. But instead of sounding like Minnie Mouse, you end up coughing like a Colorado bong-a-thon attendee. Coughing is encouraged and will open up your lungs, so let it rip.

MACHINES THAT BEEP

In the hospital, machines continuously monitor things like your breathing, pulse, fluid intake, and blood pressure. The machines, which are attached to you, click, swish, and beep while they are working fine. These same machines also beep when there is a problem. While this could cause confusion, the alarm beeps are louder and more frequent than the "I'm working okay" beeps. The alarm beeps can go off for major or minor issues, like when you move your arm a certain way or get out of bed, or an IV pump runs low on hydrating solution.

While you might be concerned about an alarm beep, the nurses, who are fluent in the language of beeps, don't always rush in to check on you. That's because they use selective hearing and may recognize that the beep is not an emergency. Or they might be tied up because every patient on your floor has pushed their call button in unison. Even if the alarm beeps drive you batty and you have deep medical knowledge from watching every season of *The Doctors*, don't try to silence the alarm yourself. Always call your nurse to deal with the alarm beeps. If your nurse doesn't respond to your call button, you can send your advocate out to the nurses' station to find a medical professional.

Moving In to the Regular Hospital Room

Hospitals are not hotels. You will not find wrapped chocolates on your pillow, six-hundred-thread-count Egyptian cotton sheets, or towels magically twisted into animal shapes. The majority of hospital rooms look like the accommodations offered by a German youth hostel—clean, stark, and simply furnished. (However, you will not have to worry about a house curfew or rowdy hostellers singing beer-drinking songs.) There is usually a telephone, a television, a bed, a chair, and a window in the hospital room. My rooms had wide-open, unobstructed views of the hospital's concrete parking garages. I could gaze out and watch drivers whip around in circles at sixty-five miles per hour, risking their lives as they vied for mattress-sized parking spaces. After witnessing this for several hours, I felt fortunate to be secure in my hospital bed, wheels locked and rails up, and tethered to an IV.

Once I was settled in my room, my nurse introduced herself and showed me how to work the electronically controlled bed, television remote, and call button. She also pointed out an emergency cord in the bathroom I could pull if I slid off the toilet. The emergency cord and call button connect to the nurses' station, where a light goes on if a patient needs help.

There are times that you should definitely use your call button, such as when you get out of bed for the first time. But it's not necessary to call the nurse to complain about the mashed potatoes from the cafeteria or that there isn't enough ice in your water. Try to let your nurse know what you need, whether it's additional blankets or to ask your doctor questions, while she is in your room checking on you. Keep a list of your requests.

If your nurse is busy with other patients and doesn't respond to your call button and it's urgent, you can send your advocate to the nurses' station to see if he can get help. Nurses work in shifts that are usually eight to twelve hours long. When the nurses are changing shifts, your nonurgent requests will need to wait. During a shift change, the outgoing nurse reviews the doctors' orders, medicines, and status for each patient with the incoming nurse. And they need to focus on this exchange of important information.

Try to be pleasant to your nurses. They want to help you get better. They can be among your best advocates in the hospital and are usually more responsive to agreeable patients. Your nurse can advise you about pain medicine or give subtle information about a doctor's skills. (If your nurse suggests getting a second opinion from another doctor, listen to her!) They can provide emotional support and share the menus of the best takeout restaurants near the hospital.

Using Pain Medicine in the Hospital

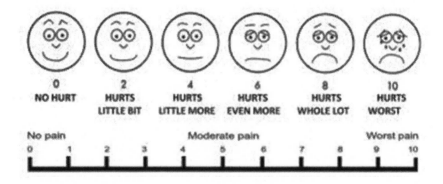

"On a scale of one to ten, what do you rate your pain at this moment in time?"

The nurses take pain control very seriously, and they will ask you this question *dozens* of times. Since pain is subjective, they give you parameters. They may hold up a pain scale that shows ten cartoon faces, from a smiling zero who has no pain at all to a weeping-in-anguish ten. Ten is the most severe pain a human can experience, such as passing a kidney stone, having natural child-birth, or stubbing your pinky toe on your new coffee table. The nurses administer drugs based on your pain number, so you want to respond to this question to the best of your ability. If you are an actuary or a former mathlete, try to rate your pain in simple whole numbers. Telling a nurse, "My current pain level is the square root of pi," or playing a math trick, such as "I'm thinking of a pain-level number between one and ten, and it's odd" will result in a delay of medication.

Right after surgery, my pain level ranged between three, as if I had just done two hundred sit-ups, and five, as if I had a bad sunburn that was going to peel no matter how much I moisturized. Since I was proactive with my morphine pump and asked for pain medicine when I hit level four or five, I never reached the dreaded eight or nine. Keep in mind that the nurses are watching your pain-related behavior; they don't want to overmedicate you. If you say you are a ten and are munching on Sun Chips, chatting about *Survivor* results on your phone, and generally acting like a two, the nurses might give you ibuprofen instead of the strong pain medicine.

Eating in the Hospital

Hospitals do not yet receive Michelin stars, but the quality and variety of the food have improved. Instead of serving mystery meat and gray gruels, my hospital's café was similar to a very mediocre Jersey diner. The menu was vast, and breakfast was available all day. I could order as much food as I wanted. If you are like my eleven-year-old son, who is offered wheat-germ muffins for breakfast at home, the hospital food will be a dream. After his elbow surgery, my son ordered puddings, milkshakes, cherry Jell-O with whipped cream, and pancakes. (No high-fructose food police patrolled his hospital cafeteria!) After eating his weight in sugar, we had no trouble getting him out of his hospital bed; he bounced off the mattress and zipped down the halls.

The first day after my surgery, I was on a clear-liquid diet, which meant I could choose to eat broth, ice chips, ginger ale, juices, popsicles, and Jell-O. Hospitals consider Jell-O a liquid food because it melts down at room temperature and is easily digested. They also believe it is the entire base of the food pyramid and will push it onto every tray leaving the cafeteria. For my first meal, I ordered a bowl of broth. Since I had not eaten in twenty hours, it was the most delicious oversalted liquid I had ever tasted. The next morning, I was allowed to resume a normal diet. Once I got my doctor's approval, I could send my advocate out for takeout or eat snacks from home.

Hospital Time

Time shrinks and stretches in the hospital. When you are under general anesthesia, three hours fly by in seconds, but time crawls when you are waiting for discharge papers. If the nurse says the doctor will be by to see you soon, soon could mean fifteen minutes or two hours. Your 10:30 surgery could be postponed until noon because the operation before yours had complications. Patient care is innately unpredictable. A surgery can go longer than expected, a lab test might need to be reprocessed or might be lost, or a fellow patient could have a medical emergency. Accept that you're on hospital time. Things might not happen as scheduled. Rather than get annoyed or stressed, try to relax and stay occupied. Read a magazine, meditate, take a nap, or watch another soothing episode of "Crafting as Therapy" on your hospital TV.

GETTING OUT OF BED AND WALKING

In order to prevent blood clots after an operation, doctors can prescribe sequential compression devices or blood-thinning medications, and they strongly encourage their patients to get up and move around. The Hospital for Special Surgery estimates that *"without* preventative care, as many as 30 to 50 percent of patients undergoing joint-replacement surgery would develop blood clots, usually in the thigh or calf."[3] But this number drops significantly with preventative care.

After my hysterectomy, I was tired and semicomfortable in my warm bed with a morphine pump and leg compressors massaging my calves. The floor looked cold, and standing up seemed like it would hurt. Since I didn't want to pull anything or disturb my stitches, I lay immobile for hours. My husband, who is a diligent advocate, repeatedly begged me to just *try* to stand up. But I felt safe in my hospital bed and didn't want to rock my boat. So instead of listening to my advocate, like I should have, I gave myself another hit from the morphine pump and floated off to dreamland.

I awoke to a nurse unplugging my compression booties and asking, "Ready to get up?" This was uttered as a statement. When I replied that I could use another nap, she insisted that I sit with my feet dangling over the edge of the bed. (Sitting is considered an activity since it requires stomach muscles.) Once I sat, she strongly encouraged me to stand. My husband and my nurse were absolutely right. I needed to get up. The sooner I started moving, the faster I reduced my blood-clot risk and began healing.

My nurse guided me out of the hospital bed with the following steps:

- She unplugged the leg compressors and IV pole and made sure the IV wasn't caught on the bed rail. The IV pole had wheels and would roll with me.
- She checked that I had on the nonslip socks that were given to me in the preoperative room. I didn't take these socks off until I got out of the hospital.
- She had me roll onto my side, push up with my arms, and lower my legs to the floor until I was sitting on the edge of the bed.
- I sat on the edge of the bed for a few minutes. The nurse turned a chair backward and placed it in front of me.
- I grabbed the top of the chair and stood for a minute. Then I held the nurse's arm until I felt balanced, and she led me and my rolling IV pole slowly to the bathroom.

Each time I got out of bed and repeated this process, it got easier. My husband helped me instead of the nurse until I was able to slide out of the bed on my own.

Preventing Falls

You want to take precautions to avoid a fall, which could extend your hospital stay. When you are in the hospital, you are on strong medication, attached to IV lines and leg compressors, and in an unfamiliar environment. Make sure to wear your nonskid socks and glasses and ask for help if you feel dizzy. Take your time getting out of bed or a chair, and check that your IV lines are out of your way. If you feel unsteady, sit right back down.

Peeing after Catheter Removal

As mentioned earlier, a urinary catheter is often used during major surgery. Once the catheter is removed, it might take a while for the urethra to relax so you can pee. It can be frustrating if you feel like you need to urinate but can't. The following tips for postcatheter peeing are based on my hospital experiences as well as witnessing the sleepover party prank of dunking a snoozing person's hand into warm water. Before you try the tinkle tips below, drink liquids to ensure that your bladder is full.

Tinkle Tips:

- Relax and visualize water images like fountains, ocean waves, and Niagara Falls.
- Turn on the faucet while you are by the toilet. The sound of running water can reduce "stage fright" and make urine flow.
- Lean forward.
- Submerge your hand in a cup of warm water and shut your eyes.
- Pour a cup of warm water slowly over your lower stomach.
- Blow bubbles with a straw into a cup of water while sitting on the toilet.

If these don't work, go back to bed, relax, drink more liquids, and try again.

Where Did My Surgeon Go?

While recovering in the hospital, the nurses, who are very capable, are your primary contacts. Your surgeon is busy performing multiple operations or having clinic hours. If you don't see much of your surgeon after your operation, that probably means you are healing fine. If you have complications, you will get more attention and visits.

My surgeons rounded, which means they checked on their hospitalized patients, early each morning between 6:00 and 8:30. I tried to be prepared for these visits with a list of questions. Have your advocate jot down questions, and take your time understanding your surgeon's answers, because you might not see her in person until your two-week post-op visit.

Who Is in Charge of Coordinating My Care in the Hospital?

While you see your nurses frequently, they are not ultimately responsible for you. The attending physician is the person who is in charge of you in the hospital. Usually it is the surgeon who performed your operation. But make sure to ask your nurse who your attending physician is. His or her name will be printed on the top of your hospital chart. The attending physician is the person you need to contact for major questions and concerns.

Keep in mind that surgeons focus on specific body parts or areas of expertise. Your orthopedic surgeon might do an excellent job on your complex knee operation but might not want to be responsible for ordering your heart medications or laxatives. Anything not directly related to your knee surgery may be covered by a hospitalist. Hospitalists are usually internal medicine doctors who only see hospitalized patients. (They don't have office hours.) There is often a team of them available twenty-four hours a day, and they know the hospital policies and doctors well. If a new medical issue comes up after your surgery, you might be referred to a hospitalist. He can help coordinate care among your doctors.

At times medicine is still practiced in silos. The doctor you see in the hospital might not be part of your primary-care physician's group; she doesn't have access to your medical history. The doctor who checks on you in a skilled nursing facility might not be able to see your surgeon's notes. You are the hub and center of your health-care team. After all, you know your body and health history better than anyone else. Your doctors and nurses are the spokes that support and care for you.

That means you and your advocate should take on the following coordination tasks:

- Ask your nurse going off duty about medicines, tests, or visits from specialists that you should receive during the next shift. When your new nurse introduces herself, check that she has this information.
- Write down what each doctor advises, any tests or procedures she recommends, and any medications she prescribes. Understand what the tests and medications are for.
- Follow up to make sure that what is supposed to happen actually happens. If necessary, track down test results, call the physical therapist if you don't hear from him, and remind the nurses you need your blood work done.
- Tell your primary-care doctor and specialists about test results and new medications you received in the hospital. Also,

communicate any new allergy information or reactions to medicines or anesthesia you experienced.

After hearing this advice, you may think, "This sounds like a lot of work. My advocate and I already have enough to deal with. Isn't there someone else who can do all this coordinating?"

There are professional patient advocates who charge a hundred dollars an hour to help coordinate care. You can find more information about them at the Alliance of Professional Health Advocates website, aphadvocates.org. But if hiring a professional is not in your budget, you and a family member will need to take on the monitoring of your health care. Think of it as volunteer work or free job training in case you ever want to embark on a career in the growing field of professional patient advocates.

Shuffling around the Hospital

The nurses wanted me to get out of bed about every two hours while I was awake. I did short two-minute walks to the bathroom, to the sink to wash my hands, or to the window to admire the parking garage. I walked in the privacy of my room when my husband was around in case I felt light-headed.

On my second day postsurgery, I left my room to do a "field trip" to the nurses' station. Before leaving my room, the nurse gave me a second hospital gown to cover up and use as a robe so I wouldn't moon people in the hallway. Since I was connected to an IV stand, a robe would have been hard to wear. I stood for two minutes holding on to the nurses' station counter before I shuffled back to bed to rest. The more you move and walk, the better you will feel.

ATTEMPTING TO SLEEP IN THE HOSPITAL

Hospitals are noisy places illuminated by four-hundred-watt fluorescent bulbs that could light up professional baseball fields or the Empire State Building. When you switch off the overhead lights, bright little lights on your monitors shine. Beeps from the medical equipment chirp throughout the day and night. Fellow patients moan. If you want to get some sleep, it's a good idea to use earplugs and an eye mask. (Once, when I forgot my earplugs, I made homemade ones with pieces of rolled-up paper towel. They can be tricky to remove. It's better to use the manufactured foam plugs.)

At night, your nurse will advise you to "rest and get some sleep." She will click off the TV and tuck in your blankets. She may adjust your pillows, get you a glass of water, and close the blinds. Your nurse will turn off the overhead lights and gently shut your door.

Then, surprise!

Your nurse will wake you up every four hours to take your temperature and pulse and inquire about your bodily functions. Night is day to her, and she is highly caffeinated. At four in the morning, she can rapidly describe her weeklong Disney vacation and then pepper you with questions about the volume and timing of your passed gas. The cleaning crew might drop by to buff your floor at five in the morning. Clearly, you will not be getting nine hours of beauty sleep. But you could get a nice four-hour stretch.

The following tips helped me and my husband, who stayed overnight on a foldout chair, get some sleep.

Tips for Sleeping in the Hospital:

* Get comfortable. Ask for extra pillows if needed. Ask your nurse for a warm blanket or to adjust the room temperature if you are too cold or hot.
* Go the bathroom.
* Mention to your nurse that you are trying to sleep. Ask if it would be possible to cluster checking your vitals with drawing your blood and cleaning your room. That way you're up only once at four in the morning.
* Ask your nurse to check that your IV bag is full, because the IV alarm will start beeping when it's low.
* Turn off the lights.
* Take a dose of pain medicine.
* Put in earplugs or earbuds to listen to soothing music or sounds. Strap on a sleep mask.
* Envision a relaxing image.

Managing Visitors

Some people in the hospital thrive on having visitors. Visitors can provide a welcome distraction and give your advocate a break. If you are in the hospital for weeks, visits and virtual visits with FaceTime or Skype can connect you to the outside world.

While I loved the idea of friends dropping by to hold my hand and feed me chocolate-covered pretzels, the reality was that I was not up for hospital visitors. I was tired, uncomfortable, and semi-naked. Rather than expend energy on chatting, I needed to save my stamina for figuring out how I was going to hoist myself out of the hospital bed.

I appreciated it when friends dropped off magazines, plants, or food to the hospital lobby. I welcomed text messages of love and concern. While in the hospital, I called my kids, sister, and mom. But talking on the phone was tiring. My husband did a good job handling phone calls, texts, and potential visitors. He told friends that I was out of it and it would be better if they checked in on me once I returned home.

If you do have visitors, your advocate can manage them. He can make sure everyone washes their hands, lead the small talk, and help open gifts. If you get tired, your advocate can suggest that you need to rest and move the visitors along. If you don't have an advocate, ask your nurses to drop by ten minutes into a visit and announce that it's time for you to rest. Or you can tell your visitors that while you enjoy seeing them, it's your nap time.

CHECKING OUT OF THE HOSPITAL

Be aware that leaving the hospital is not like checking out of the Hyatt. The discharge process is often delayed; you could be sitting around for hours waiting for test results, medications, wheelchair transportation, and written instructions. Before leaving the hospital, I needed to meet my doctor's criteria for discharge, which included eating, drinking, and using the toilet on my own. Discharge criteria will depend on your doctor and type of surgery.

Once the nurse had a written order of discharge from the doctor, she gave me a sheet of typed instructions. The instructions detailed my medications, when I could drive again and resume other activities, and when to call the doctor. (I was supposed to call if I had a fever over 101, severe pain, vomiting, redness or pus at the incision site, or shortness of breath.)

I received pages of detailed discharge information. Since I was groggy, it was good to have my advocate there to review the instructions with the nurse. He kept asking questions until he was clear on everything. You want to make sure that your advocate understands your discharge orders. (If you have a home visit from a nurse, she can also re-review the discharge instructions with you when you are situated at home.)

If you are going home with medical devices such as drains, a spirometer, or an oxygen tank, make sure you and your advocate understand how to use them. Do a demonstration for the discharge nurse. Ask her to recommend some medical websites where you can view videos of how to use your medical equipment. Understand how often you need to use your device and how to clean it.

The following are discharge questions you should get answered before checking out.

* How long do I take my prescription meds for? Do I take them with food, and how often? (See Medicine Review, below.)
* Can I go home and eat whatever I want? Do I have any dietary restrictions? When can I start taking my usual vitamins and supplements?
* When can I resume driving? How long until I can lean over and lift more than five or ten pounds?
* Do I have to change my bandages or can I just leave them alone? Can I take a shower with the bandages on?

* Is there any kind of follow-up physical therapy to this surgery or special exercises I should do? How much walking should I be doing during my recovery?
* How many days after surgery should I have a follow-up appointment with the doctor? Has the appointment been scheduled?
* What are some things I should look out for? Do I call you if I have a fever, vomiting, or shortness of breath?
* If I am taking home medical equipment like drains or a walker, could you show me how to use them?
* Can we do a medicine review of all my prescription and over-the-counter drugs?

Do a Medicine Review with a Nurse

After an operation, you will receive several new prescriptions. Before you leave the hospital, you and your advocate need to go over each prescription with a nurse so you know what you are taking, why you are taking it, when to take it, how to take it, and for how long you should take it.

You can draft a chart like the one on the next page. (There is a blank chart at the end of this book.) After you understand how your new prescriptions will be taken, review the medicines, vitamins, and supplements that you were on *before* surgery to determine what you can and cannot take during recovery. For example, your doctor might want you to continue to take your calcium pills right after surgery but hold off on the baby aspirin and fish oil, which can thin your blood. Call your pharmacist or doctor if you have any questions about medicines, doses, drug interactions, or reactions.

A medication can have several names, which can be confusing. There can be a catchy brand name, like Advil, and a hard-to-pronounce generic name, like ibuprofen. (The generic names often sound like inhospitable Star Wars planets.) The brand names are created by marketing whizzes who want to entice you to buy cases of their product. The generic name is a shorthand of a drug's chemical components and structure as identified by methodical chemists.[4] Write down both names on your chart. Keep in mind that generic drugs, which are usually just as effective as brand-name drugs, can be much cheaper.

EXAMPLE OF A MEDICATION CHART

Note: This chart can be updated throughout your recovery as you move from the stronger prescribed drugs to over-the-counter pain meds.

Drug name (brand and generic)	What does this drug do? Why am I taking it?	Dose and color of pill	When to take it/with or without food?	Date/Time Taken
Ibuprofen, (brand name: Advil)	Pain control/fever reducer	200mg, dark rose color	One tablet every 4-6 hours, with food	11/9 One tablet at 8 am One tablet at 1 pm
Ranitidine (brand name: Zantac)	Heartburn relief	75 mg, pink color with a Z	Take two tablets with a glass of water. Can be used up to twice daily	11/9 One tablet at 7 am
Oxycodone-Acetaminophen (brand name: Percocet)	Pain Control	Oxycodone Hydrochloride, USP 7.5 mg Acetaminophen, USP 325 mg, white color	Take one tablet by mouth every six hours as needed.	11/9 One tablet at 6 am

The Drive Home

Before you leave the hospital, ask your nurses for pain and (if needed) nausea medication for the ride home. Make sure you have enough pain medication to tide you over until you can get your prescriptions filled at your local pharmacy.

Once I received my discharge information, I took a dose of pain medicine. My husband retrieved our car, and I was taken in a wheelchair to the lobby. (If you had anesthesia, a narcotic, or a muscle relaxant like Valium, you will *not* be allowed to drive yourself home from inpatient or outpatient surgery.) I slid into my minivan, with its low seats, and stuck a small travel pillow between my seat belt and the stitches on my stomach. I didn't want the seat belt to rub against my incision. If I held the pillow against my stomach, the bumps on the road didn't bother me.

If you have a long drive, try to get out and stretch your legs every hour or so to decrease the risk of blood clots. Point and flex your toes and move your feet in circles to keep your blood flowing.

CHAPTER 9

Recovering at Home

◆ ◆ ◆

WELCOME HOME! YOU MADE IT over the mountain of surgery and are heading down the recovery slope. The "ding, ding, ding" sounds from medical machines are fading into the past. You'll be able to eat, rest, and sleep better now that you are home.

The first thing I did after inching up the steps to my house and shuffling through the front door was to go directly to bed. My care-taker left a glass of water, a snack, and my cell phone and charger on my bedside table. He lined up my pain medications on a nearby dresser. It was comforting to see that the pain pills would be right there when I needed them.

MANAGING PAIN AND MEDICINES AT HOME

The discharge nurse reminded me that pain management would help my body to heal. I needed to "stay ahead of the pain" at home. This meant taking prescription pain medications as di-rected as well using extra-strength Advil (ibuprofen) and Tylenol (acetaminophen). Some pain medications were to be taken every four hours, others every six hours, and some were taken as need-ed. I kept a medication schedule on a pad of paper next to my drugs. Some patients use their cell phone alarms to track their medications. There are also free phone apps like Medisafe that send audible reminders to take your medicine and track when you last took it.

During the first four to five days postsurgery, I relied on my prescription pain medicine. Before bed, I set my phone alarm to ring for my middle-of-the-night dose. After about five days, I moved to the maximum dose of extra-strength Tylenol during the day and took the strong prescription painkillers only before bed. Eventually, I was using the Advil and Tylenol on an as-needed basis.

If you have nausea from your medications, you can try taking your pills after a meal. You can also call your doctor and ask for a different pain medication. Another possibility is to eat bland food like toast, crackers, and bananas for a day or two to see if that helps your stomach.

FUZZY MED HEAD

Strong prescription pain medications can make you forgetful and spacey during your recovery. (This is not the time to host important work conference calls or try to beat the stock market.) During my recuperation, I would think of something very important that I needed to do the in the kitchen. Usually, it was to see if we had run out of milk, which in my house disappears at an alarming rate of five gallons per week. (Where does it all go? I suspect cover-ups of multiple milk spills and secret chugging contests are occurring.) By the time I got off the couch and shuffled to the kitchen, the very important thing floated out of my mind. No matter how many times

I thought, "There is something I need to do in here. Did it start with an A?" my mind remained blank as I went through the alphabet.

After this happened several times, I started sending reminder texts to myself before I left the couch. I would take my phone with me and read the text when I arrived in the kitchen. If there was something really important, I wrote it on my hand. For things that I needed to do every day, I stuck Post-its on the fridge or set reminders on my phone. If I was reading a book with multiple characters, I wrote down who the characters were on a sheet of paper and stuck the paper in the book. As I moved from the prescription opioids to Tylenol, my focus and memory improved.

Managing Your Incisions and Medical Devices at Home

If you are sent home with a medical device like a spirometer, drains, or an oxygen tank, use the device exactly as prescribed. Review the written instructions you received from the discharge nurse. Make sure to keep medical devices away from pets and children. Follow safety information. If you are using oxygen, take extra precautions, like keeping the canister five to ten feet away from open flames, including candles and gas stovetops.

Once you are home, call your nurse if you have any questions. She may be able to direct you to some hospital websites that have pictures or videos of how to use your medical device. If you have an upcoming appointment and still have some questions, you can bring the medical equipment with you to show the nurse how you have been using it.

As far as taking care of your incisions, follow your doctor's instructions about changing the dressing and keeping the area dry. Doctors don't want you to use ointments or lotions on your stitches or to remove the dressing until they tell you to. It's normal to have some soreness, itching, bruising, or numbness around the incision. It's *not* normal to have an incision that feels hot, has a red surrounding area, or has a yellow or green discharge. These could be signs of an infection, and you should call your doctor.

My incisions were closed with stitches that looked like stiff black threads. The stitches were covered with white strips of tape, called Steri-Strips. Gauze (also known as "dressing") was taped over the Steri-Strips. I was told not to touch the dressing or stitches until my postsurgery appointment, which was ten days after my operation. The stitches would dissolve on their own in a few weeks. The nurse mentioned that I might feel strange twinges and "zaps" as things healed, and that was normal. After a few weeks, the stitches turned a lumpy red. After about five months, they started flattening and fading into white lines. It can take up to a year for a scar to finish healing.

RESTING AT HOME

After major surgery, your body needs to repair itself with sleep and rest. As mentioned earlier, resting is relaxing with your feet up. Watching TV, reading, and listening to music while lying horizontally are examples of resting. Eating, walking to the bathroom, and showering are considered activities. It's a good idea to alternate between rest and activity. Continue taking short, periodic walks; it will help speed up your recovery.

During my recovery, I fully committed myself to following my doctors' advice to take it easy. Since I was a slow healer and my body took longer to recover than the average patient, I became an expert at resting and lying around. But I also tried to get up and move frequently between rest periods.

My daily schedule early in my recovery looked like this:

<u>7:30 a.m.</u>: Sit on edge of bed. Take pain medication. Slide back under the covers until pain meds hit.

<u>8:15–8:28 a.m.</u>: Shuffle to the kitchen and do four slow laps around the breakfast table. Chat with my kids as they eat their Cheerios and make their own lunches. They are picked up by a neighbor to go to school.

<u>8:30–10:00 a.m.</u>: Go back to bed. Read. Gather my mental strength to motivate myself to get up and shower.

<u>10:00–10:06 a.m.</u>: Shower.

<u>10:07–11:35 a.m.</u>: Recover from showering. Lie flat on my living room couch. Stare at a medium-sized chip in our recessed ceiling. Try to remember if anyone recently threw a hard bouncy ball or shoe at the ceiling. Listen to the mysterious popping and creaking noises my house makes.

<u>11:40 a.m.–12:00 noon</u>: Google ghosts.

<u>12:00 noon–12:15 p.m.</u>: Shuffle around the house, find pepper spray, and check that the doors are locked. End up in kitchen eating a turkey sandwich and a Vicodin.

<u>12:18–12:45 p.m.</u>: Explore ceiling repairs on Pinterest. Become dizzy and exhausted from looking at photos of perfect ceilings from a thousand angles.

<u>12:46–2:00 p.m.</u>: Post-Pinteresting nap.

<u>2:02–2:10 p.m.</u>: Take slow laps around the living room. Hum "Eye of the Tiger."

<u>2:11–3:45 p.m.</u>: (Return to the couch.) Watch *Ellen* while texting a heroic friend who recently donated a kidney to her brother. Ponder what it would be like to save someone's life. (See DonateLife.net to find out.)

<u>3:50–4:10 p.m.</u>: Get up to eat another turkey sandwich and left-over lasagna. Let kids in from school. Enjoy hearing about their day. But start to feel achy.

<u>4:11–6:00 p.m.</u>: Get back on the couch. (No surprise there.) Pop a Tylenol. Interact with my children using the minimum amount of movement and speech. Encourage my youngest to give me a foot massage in her Orbeez soothing foot spa to keep her busy. Then let her paint my toenails whatever color she wants.

<u>6:00–7:15 p.m.</u>: Wonder husband comes home and heats up dinner, serves it, gets kids to clean up and feed the dog, and supervises the laundry process while answering work e-mails and analyzing the minute but significant nuances of Monday Night Football.

<u>7:15–7:40 p.m.</u>: Help my children with their homework while resting in bed. Accept that my eighth grader's algebra is beyond my comprehension. Gently explain that they teach math very, very

differently now and that she needs to google Khan Academy for the rest of her schooling.

7:41 p.m.: Achy. Take prescription pain meds. Tsunami of tiredness. Fall into a deep sleep before my third grader, the entire population of Spain (the land of the eleven o'clock dinner), and Bert and Ernie.

MOVING SLOWLY AND PROTECTING YOUR INCISION

After your operation, you will not be moving at top speed. You might feel vulnerable and cautious. These are common feelings and to be expected. After all, you just had major surgery. Leave extra time to travel to appointments.

When I went to the hospital for my post-hysterectomy checkup, I moved at sloth speed. I didn't want to jiggle my sore stitches or bump into anything. It was the first time I had left the house in ten days, and I hunched protectively over my stomach. While taking tentative baby steps into the busy hospital lobby, I looked up to see people motoring toward me and speeding past me. My first thought, as I held my arm out to block my stomach, was "I am going to get mowed down." (I later learned that the unofficial hospital corridor etiquette is to pass on the left. The slowest walkers, including people like me who suddenly stop and don't move for periods of time, should be hugging the right wall.)

As I inched through the hospital lobby, I heard pitter-patter steps, and a toddler in pigtails passed me. Then a gray-haired lady with a black cane thumped by. By the time I got to my surgeon's office, I had been passed by texting walkers; nine-months-pregnant walkers; child walkers; ancient, withered walkers; walkers with crutches;

knee-scooter walkers; and walkers using walkers. And that was okay! The important thing was that I made it to the reception area under my own volition. When a speedy nurse lost me twice as I followed her to a distant examination room and then backtracked and exclaimed loudly, "Oh, there you are!," it was fine! Instead of shivering on the exam table in a gown and wondering if the nurses had forgotten about me, I arrived at my examination room *at the same time as my doctor.* A first! Most importantly, my checkup went well.

And in a few weeks, my walking speed returned to normal.

Grooming during Recovery

People, especially women, sometimes pressure themselves to look perfect. But in life, unless you are Kate Middleton or some other royal promoting your country's fashion designers, it is not your duty to be immaculately dressed, made up, and coifed at all times. (We are fine just as we are in our almost-fitting jeans.) This is never truer than after an operation or hospitalization, when you have limited strength. During this time, it is your job to follow your doctor's instructions, which includes getting plenty of rest.

Many patients embrace the fresh-faced look during their recovery. Perhaps they read the influential *Cosmopolitan* article "I Didn't Wear Makeup for a Week and My Skin Never Looked Better." Or maybe they would rather spend their energy watching Netflix and prying open a pint of Ben and Jerry's than examining themselves in the mirror. Other people feel naked without fixing their faces and bring a makeup bag the size of a Goldendoodle to the hospital. They say they feel better when they look better. When you are really fatigued, you pick and choose how you spend your energy.

The choice that worked for me was to look worse to feel better. During the first two weeks of recovery, I couldn't lift the hair dryer or lean over to wash my face. Using a grabber to pull on a clean pair of socks was an accomplishment. I was narcotized and housebound and had no interest in applying makeup or removing the scrunchie that was growing into my scalp. The skin around my stitches was bruised and puffy, and I wasn't allowed to shower for days. The less I focused on my physical appearance, the better I felt. While I was not looking my best, I was relieved to be through surgery and busy consuming turkey sandwiches and arranging myself on the couch.

I did feel a tiny twinge of concern for the doctors who examined me in this postoperative state. But be assured, it's impossible to gross out doctors. One of the required classes in medical school, which involves highly unattractive views of the human body, is called Gross Anatomy. By the time medical students are real doctors, they have been completely desensitized to blood, guts, smells, and any other thing your body can dish out. Doctors see the human anatomy as endlessly fascinating, and its unusual presentations are learning opportunities.

RECOGNIZING INTERNAL STITCHES AND LISTENING TO YOUR BODY

After my first major surgery, there were three small areas of external stitches on my stomach that healed in about three weeks. What I couldn't see were the hundreds of deep internal stitches that took longer to heal. These internal stitches, which were eventually absorbed by my body, are what required a six-week recovery. I did not want my internal stitches to tear loose or for adhesions to form. (Adhesions are formed by internal scar tissue that can stick organs together, which might need to be unstuck with surgery.) So my motto for any activity I wasn't sure I should do was "If in doubt, leave it out until I check it out (with my nurse or doctor)."

I tried to listen to my body. If I felt a sharp pain in my stomach when pulling wet clothes out of the washing machine, I stopped lifting immediately. If I was sore after going to the supermarket in the morning, I spent the afternoon resting.

Besides listening to my body, I tried to listen to the little voice inside my head. If I started a new activity, such as taking my muscular dog, Mickey, for a walk, and the little voice, which sounded like Marge Simpson, said, "This may not be a good idea. What if Mickey spots his archnemesis, our friendly UPS man? Mickey will go berserk and yank me into the big brown truck as he lunges for the UPS man's nether regions," I listened to the little voice and waited before walking my dog. There was plenty of time in the future to exercise my pet, but I only had one chance to heal.

WHAT IF I FEEL GREAT BUT MY DOCTOR SAYS I NEED TO REST?

Some people are fast healers and are in tremendous physical condition going into surgery. During their recovery, they listen to their bodies as their doctors advised, and their bodies holler, "Sprint out the front door, jog to the gym, and give me fifty squats!" But before you do this, you need to ask yourself the following questions:

* Do I have internal stitches that need time to heal?
* Am I following my medical team's instructions about what I can and cannot do during recovery?

* Has my doctor seen me and cleared me for exercise?
* Am I on a drug high?

Think about the answers to these questions. If you are too active too soon, you could delay healing by stressing the stitches or causing scar tissue to form where it shouldn't. Check in with your medical team and get their opinion about what level of exercise and activity is appropriate for you.

Moving and Exercising during Recovery: Why Should I Bother?

Your postsurgery activity plan might include physical therapy, walking, and specific exercises and stretches.

Some of the benefits of exercising, which can include just walking, are the following:

* It will improve your circulation.
* It can help you sleep better and have a better appetite.
* It will improve your mood and decrease the postsurgery blues.
* You'll heal faster and have a faster recovery.
* It can help your immune system.

For my six-week recovery from a hysterectomy, I was banned from jogging, swimming, running, biking, lifting more than five to ten pounds, or zumbaing for six weeks. I did not have physical therapy but was instructed to gradually increase my amount of walking each week.

Here are some general tips for postsurgery exercise:

- Ask your medical team for exercise guidance. How much can you do when? What type of exercise can you do?
- Start out slowly, go at your own pace, and gradually increase the amount of exercise.
- Wear comfortable shoes and clothes, and walk on flat surfaces.
- Plan to rest after exercise.
- Cut back on your speed and distance if you feel uncomfortable or exhausted.
- Bring your cell phone with you if you are walking alone.

A Walking Plan

Everyone recovers at his or her own pace. Recovery can depend on the type of surgery you have, your fitness level going into surgery, and how well your surgery goes. My postsurgery walking goal was to increase my walking time approximately five minutes each week until I could walk thirty minutes continuously by six weeks after surgery. (This goal was based on asking a nurse specific recovery questions.)

I counted meandering to the bathroom or kitchen as a two-minute walk. My walks during the second and third weeks consisted of small laps around the interior of my house. Walking to appointments or while doing errands counted toward daily goals.

Walking Plan: Goal is to walk 30 minutes continuously by week 6 post surgery		
Recovery Week	**Minutes**	**Times per day**
1	2-3	4-6
2	4-10	3-4
3	10-15	3-4
4	15-20	2-3
5	20-25	1-2
6	25-30	1
7 and on	30-35	1

MANAGING FATIGUE

Fatigue can last for weeks after surgery. It's normal. Two months past major surgery, I could drop to my couch and sleep for twelve hours. This would happen after a long walk or at seven o'clock when my kids and dog were starving for dinner. When fatigue rolls in, acknowledge it. Sit down, put your feet up, take a nap, or go to bed.

It can be hard for your family to understand your limited energy. I tried to explain to my children how I was managing my stamina using our favorite crunchy-wafer vanilla Power Bars. I laid out the delicious, addictive bars on the kitchen table and said something like this: "Mom starts each day with four vanilla Power Bars, representing four blocks of energy. Every activity or outing eats away at my bars. A morning of grocery shopping could take three Power Bars. A meeting at school later the same day uses three more Power Bars. Six Power Bars are over my daily limit of four. So I'll need to move my activities to different days or borrow Power Bars from the next day, which means resting for a chunk of time." (This little speech was interrupted several times as my children tried to eat the Power Bars.) Another possibility would be to downshift an activity into something that requires less energy. I could call in to the school meeting instead of being there in person or shop for groceries online and have them delivered.

The following are **fatigue management tips** that helped me:

* While it is early in your recovery, schedule just one outing a day. Plan to rest after the outing.
* I had more energy in the mornings, so I would run my errands then. Plus, the stores were less crowded in the morning.
* Sit instead of standing. Sit on your bed while getting dressed. Sit while waiting to be seated at a restaurant. Sit while watching your kid's soccer games.
* Call or Skype in to meetings.
* If you are out and feel exhausted, leave and go home.
* Drink plenty of water, eat well, exercise, and sleep.
* Plan how to use your energy. If you have an important event at seven o'clock at night, take a late nap and take it easy during the day.
* Ask for help at stores. Two grocery-bagging professionals assured me that they enjoyed going outside in the fresh air to push carts and load bags into cars.
* Don't stay up late for TV shows; record them. Use the TV as a babysitter so you can rest.

STAYING POSITIVE DURING YOUR RECOVERY

Recovery isn't linear. While recuperating from major surgery, there might be days when you feel almost normal and times when you feel like a washed-up weakling. The first four to five days postsurgery are the toughest. I found that my postoperative blues depended on how long I was under anesthesia, my pain level, my medications, and my physical and mental states going into surgery. When I had an operation after two weeks of partial bed rest, it was a longer haul than when I went into a surgery in decent physical shape.

What helped me get through the postoperative blues was to bribe myself into a healing cycle. If I was physically active, my appetite increased and I slept better at night. Sleeping well at night improved my mood. If I was rested and in a better mood, it was easier to increase my walking and activity levels. To get a jump-start on this, I used rewards. I watched an engrossing TV show after doing ten minutes of walking. Other motivational treats could be shopping online while in bed or making a homemade Coolatta with ice cream and coffee.

Major surgery or a serious illness affects how we look at life. It can uncover our hidden strengths, make us appreciative, and help us focus on how we spend our time. These insights are sometimes referred to as the "gift of surgery." While l would have preferred to return this gift for a refund or exchange it for a Vitamix, writing down the positive things I learned made me feel productive. (You will develop your own surgery insights, but feel free to borrow any of the following.)

INSIGHTS FROM SURGERY AND RECOVERY

* Worrying about your health doesn't protect you from illness or prepare you for surgery. As a healing hypochondriac, I worry less and pay more attention to what is going on right now in front of my face.

- You don't know what you can get through until you have to get through it. And then you just wade through it.
- I am good at napping.
- Visualizing and planning a postrecovery family trip to New Orleans helped me through the down days.
- There is nothing like medical bed rest to make you appreciate walking to the mailbox.
- I enjoy consuming hot, cold, and lukewarm lasagna and can contentedly eat it for four consecutive meals.
- EMTs, doctors, and nurses make surgery and saving lives seem easy. I am extremely grateful that they do their jobs so well.
- My kids are helpful and resilient and much better at making waffles than I am.
- I can say no. When you have limited energy, you choose the activities that are enjoyable or important to *you*. I no longer just go with the flow; I stop and evaluate. After my surgeries, I resigned from a nonprofit board. I weighed the required time commitment against my contributions and personal fulfillment and decided to leave. I said no to an extended family trip that involved flying on small planes to a cold, mountainous place. Everyone else was welcome to go, I explained, but I don't like small planes, the cold, or the mountains. I wouldn't be taking the trip.
- No matter how wonderful your spouse and friends are, they aren't mind readers or responsible for your happiness. Be your own booster. If moo shu pork with hoisin sauce and thin pancakes makes me happy, but the vast majority of my friends and family dislike Chinese food, I now make a lunch date with myself. I order up the moo shu and enjoy each pancake.

Besides writing down what I learned from surgery, I found escapism and distraction to be helpful tools for getting through a recovery.

* **Escape through planning.** Plan a trip. Plan an outing or a party. You don't necessarily have to go on the trip or host the gathering; the planning process is a positive distraction. During my recovery, I spent two enjoyable days researching European family river cruises—and their associated excursions—on which I will probably never set sail. My husband gets seasick and, as a rule of thumb, we avoid "culturally enriching excursions to quaint European historic towns" with our children. (We have learned through trial and error to only expose them to beach or amusement-park cultures.) But I enjoyed studying the river cruise passenger reviews, sample menus, and itineraries.
* **Escape through movies and books.** Read or watch *Game of Thrones, The Crown, Outlander,* a Ken Follett or Sarah Haas series, or whatever escapist material transports you to a different realm or world.
* **Visit websites or look at videos that make you laugh.** Check out The Onion's or Cracked's websites and *Saturday Night Live* or Monty Python skits on YouTube.
* **Try something new.** Play a new video game or a phone app like Words with Friends to take your mind off your recovery. Try takeout from a new restaurant or watch a movie on a topic you know nothing about.

Here are some other ideas to keep you sane during your recovery:

* **Make a new connection.** Ask your medical providers for names of online support groups for people with your medical condition.

- **Go outside.**
- **Celebrate recovery goals.** The first time you take a shower on your own, get your stitches out, or drive, congratulate and treat yourself.
- **Plan something to look forward to each day.**
  - Watch a favorite TV episode.
  - Call or text a friend.
  - Read an absorbing book or magazine.

SETTING RECOVERY GOALS

For some surgeries, your medical team might give you specific daily or weekly recovery goals. Your nurse might advise that you should be off your crutches two weeks after anterior cruciate ligament (ACL) surgery. Your occupational therapist can set a goal for you to shower unassisted by day seven after your operation.

For my surgeries, I was given general recovery guidelines. I was told that I could probably to go back to work six weeks after my operation, depending on how I healed. During my first surgery, I worked part time from home selling camp-registration software. It wasn't clear to me how in six weeks I was going to get from point A, spending ten hours a day drug addled on the couch, to point B, enthusiastically selling and demonstrating summer-camp online applications. In order to make my big recovery goals, I needed to break them into small steps.

Besides returning to work, I had two other long-term goals. One was to play tennis again, and the other was to attend my eighth grader's back-to-school night, which would involve navigating the labyrinth of her middle school and finding six different teachers' rooms. The layout of our middle school remains a deep mystery. This is due to the building design and the students, who beg parents to keep two miles away from school property at all times. Once you turn twelve, everything a parent does, including standing, breathing, and blinking on school grounds, is horribly embarrassing. Back-to-school night was my small window of opportunity to enter the school, meet the teachers, and donate to the PTO in person in exchange for a release from future coupon-book fund-raisers.

But your goals might be different from mine. If you are working with a physical therapist, she can help you set specific, realistic goals and a path to reach them. Since I did not have a physical therapist, I relied on my medical team for general recovery guidelines. I also reviewed a helpful website called Hystersisters.com for recovery milestones. I then drafted some weekly goals that I reviewed with a nurse, who said they were acceptable.

Recovery Goals after Surgery Chart

Long Term Recovery Goals	Weekly Goals	Daily Goals
Return to work six weeks after operation	*Weeks 1-2*: Get out of bed on my own, practice sitting in a chair, walk five minutes more each week	Sit in a chair for 15 minutes, take four short walks a day
Attend back-to-school night six weeks after operation	*Weeks 3-4:* Move from prescription pain meds to ibuprofen, continue to increase walking time by five minutes a week	Take two 10-15 minute walks per day, sit for 30 minutes at a time several times a day
	Weeks 5-6: Start driving, walk a mile in the park, go out for coffee or lunch with a friend	Do one errand every day, continue walking plan
Play tennis six months after operation	*Weeks 1-6:* Complete the goals above	Complete daily goals above
	Weeks 7-12: Speed walk for 15 minutes	Speed walk for 15 minutes as part of daily 30-minute walk
	Weeks 13-20: Light jogging for 10 minutes	Light jog for 5-10 minutes as part of daily 30-minute walk
	Weeks 21-26: Play tennis for 15-30 minutes with an understanding, noncompetitive friend	

Rewarding Yourself

Having rewards and celebrating recovery milestones kept me motivated. Big milestones like driving and taking a hot shower unassisted were rewards in themselves. Small treats also helped. After increasing my walking time to fifteen minutes, I watched three episodes of *Downton Abbey*. After my first post-op appointment, my husband picked up food from our favorite restaurant.

It doesn't matter what the reward is as long as it's in your budget, motivates you, and is legal. The following list may give you some ideas.

* Song from iTunes
* Movie, TV show, podcast, or book
* Fancy coffee or tea from Starbucks or Teavana
* Mani-pedi or spa treatment
* Takeout from your favorite restaurant
* Charm necklace or bracelet (you can add charms as you achieve recovery milestones)
* Tickets to a professional or college basketball game or another sporting event
* Rereading your favorite book
* A hearty plant
* Concert tickets
* Going out to dinner or brunch
* Favorite juice-bar smoothie
* Hiding out in a quiet room of your local library and perusing fashion or sports magazines
* A chunk of chocolate
* Exercise clothing or sports gear—after reaching a walking goal of twenty minutes, I treated myself to parachute exercise pants

RETURNING TO WORK

Many people start back to work on a part-time basis after surgery and gradually increase their hours. If you have a physical job that involves heavy lifting or extensive driving, you will need more time off than someone who does computer work. Also, if you had complications or other health issues, you might need more time. You could ask to start back by working from home a few half-days a week. Discuss your return-to-work plan with your surgeon and get her input and approval. During your first week back at the office, you might want to plan time to rest when you get home from work.

If your boss pressures you to come back to the office but your doctor hasn't cleared you to return to work, you can tell your boss that you plan to follow your doctor's orders. It doesn't matter if your supervisor's mom returned to work two weeks after her knee-replacement surgery; you need to do what your doctor recommends for your knee replacement. While it's flattering to be needed at work, you don't want to go back until you are physically ready.

Since I was the least successful salesperson on my team, my boss did not pressure me to return work. "Absolutely do *not* push yourself! Take *all* the time in the world you need," she repeatedly reassured me. (My absence improved her sales productivity ratios.) I ended up going back to work nine weeks after my surgery. When I finally returned, I made my sales phone calls in the morning in bed and took copious notes. The notes helped me remember conversations and what I needed to follow up on or communicate to my boss. At first, I could only sit in front of the computer, on a donut pillow, for two hours at a time. (The donut pillow is a padded circle that mysteriously supports your innards.) But I gradually built up my endurance over the next month.

TRAVELING AFTER SURGERY

Anytime you are confined in a seat for long periods of time, you have an increased risk of blood clots. After an operation, your body tries to protect injured tissues and keep you from bleeding too much. For two to three months after major surgery, there is an increased risk of blood clots, or deep vein thrombosis. If a clot forms in the deep veins, such as the ones in your thigh, the clot can become large and break free and travel to the lungs.[1]

If you decide to take a long trip by plane, car, bus, or train during your recovery, check with your doctor before you make plans. Ask your doctor's opinion about taking the trip and if she has any specific recommendations for you. You might want to travel with a companion, who can act as your personal valet and help carry heavy bags and remind you to get up and move around.

LONG CAR TRIPS AFTER SURGERY

About two months after a surgery, I took an eight-hour car trip to Florida with my family. While sitting in the passenger seat and drinking lots of water, I avoided crossing my legs. In order to reduce the risk of a blood clot, I pointed and flexed my toes, moved my legs in circles, and wore knee-high compression socks. (Compression tube socks can be purchased from Amazon and hidden under jeans or worn with shorts and skirts, where they provide a youthful Catholic-schoolgirl look a la Mary Katherine Gallagher.)

Most importantly, we stopped about every two hours so I could improve my circulation by walking around our parked car for three to five minutes. Unfortunately, my husband and children, who are genetically blessed with watermelon-size bladders, hate to stop on car trips. They viewed our eight-hour drive to the Florida panhandle as the *Amazing Race*; each rest stop could get us eliminated or, worse, reduce our beach time. But my four walking breaks at Alabama gas stations not only improved my circulation; they were an opportunity for the kids to experience a slice of Americana. This included sampling pork barbecued on a spit inside the gas station, viewing crimson "BAMA" undergarments, and perusing aisles of high-powered fireworks that could easily blow the service station and our minivan directly to the sugar-white Gulf beaches. These stops ended up being a win-win: it was good for everyone's health to get up and stretch, and the barbecue sandwiches were delicious.

Long Plane Trips after Surgery

When taking a long plane ride, it's a good idea to get up and stretch and stroll about every two hours. This could be a challenge if you are on a bumpy flight or if you are like me and need a Valium, Xanax, or margarita in a large, unmarked to-go cup to enter an airplane cabin. Unfortunately, after surgery, we need to limit the use of sleeping pills, sedative drugs, and liquid courage when taking long flights. That's because, while catnaps are fine, you don't want to pass out into a deep four- or five-hour sleep.

The following are tips for reducing the risk of a blood clot during a long flight:

- Stand, stretch, and walk in the airport before your flight takes off. The TSA makes this easy! Standing in winding security lines, stretching your hands above your head to be scanned with invisible rays, and undergoing intimate pat-downs will improve your circulation and blood flow.
- Sit in an aisle seat so you can easily get up to stretch and walk.
- Drink water, not vodka.
- Wear compression socks or compression stockings.

* When sitting, point and flex your toes and move your feet off the floor.

* It's helpful to be seated next to a "sensitive" baby or in front of a toddler who kicks your seat back to the beat of his Wiggles CD. Their presence will drive you to a distant part of the plane. If the flight attendants ask why you're hanging out in the narrow aisles, explain that you are following your doctor's orders for your medical condition. Offer to pass out the pretzels.

PHYSICAL THERAPY

Physical therapy can be an important part of recovery. Depending on the type of surgery you have, the nurses might show you some basic physical therapy exercises in the hospital that you can start right away. But not all surgery requires physical therapy. For gynecological and gallbladder recoveries, therapy can be just walking. For knee- or hip-replacement surgery, physical therapy is critical in getting your mobility back. The doctor writes a prescription for a specific number of sessions with a physical therapist. Ask your nurse or doctor for recommendations of good physical therapists who have experience with your type of recovery.

Sometimes physical therapists will make house calls, but usually you go to their office, which looks like a health club. Physical therapists are known as the cool kids of the medical world. They are often attractive, in great shape, and outgoing. Your insurance company pays for them to stretch and rub your body parts. (Don't overthink this. Enjoy!) Keep in mind that insurance companies might cover a set number of therapy sessions with in-network therapists. Check with your insurance company to see how many sessions it will pay for.

Think of your physical therapist as your personal trainer. Tell her about your goals, whether it's to play golf again or to go hiking. Tell her if something hurts. Ask questions. Make sure you understand how to do the exercises that she gives for homework and how often you are supposed to do them.

After my son's elbow surgery, his surgeon prescribed two months of physical therapy to improve his arm's range of motion. (Range of motion is how far a joint like an elbow or knee can flex and extend. An elbow can lack ten degrees of full extension due to surgery.) My son was scheduled for two half-hour sessions per week. While we had been cautiously protecting his elbow, his physical therapist had no qualms about grabbing it, stretching it, and smushing it against the table. (The stretching and smushing were intense, but significantly improved his arm's range of motion.) The physical therapist also led my son through strengthening exercises using giant rubber bands and weights. At the end of the session, my son was covered in a massive ice pack and given a printout of homework exercises. The more often he did the exercises, the faster he regained his range of motion.

OVERVIEW OF A POSTOPERATIVE DOCTOR'S APPOINTMENT

My postoperative doctor's appointment took place about ten days after surgery. I wasn't cleared for driving, so a family member drove me to the appointment. Since I was moving at sloth speed, I gave myself extra time to brush my teeth, get to the car, and shuffle into the doctor's office. My family member carried my purse and my list of questions for the doctor.

I popped Tylenol about an hour before the appointment, just in case I was going to get an invasive exam. (At this point in my recovery, I did not want to be touched anywhere below my earlobes without being medicated.) My appointment began with a nurse weighing me and taking my blood pressure and temperature. Then I met with my surgeon. She asked about how I was feeling, if I had any fevers, and the frequency of my bowel movements. (Doctors have a deep and profound medical interest in poop.) The answers to these questions helped steer the direction of the exam. The doctor looked at my external incisions and gently poked them. I got out my list of questions about what activities I should or should not be doing. I also asked for a copy of my surgery reports to keep in my big black binder. The appointment lasted about fifteen minutes.

CAREGIVERS NEED CARE

While it's important to take care of yourself during recovery, let's not forget about the supportive person who doles out your medicine, fixes your meals, and takes you to the doctor. Your caregiver could be balancing work and other commitments while nursing you back to health. Some people thrive on nursing a loved one and relish their role; for others it's a challenge. In order to avoid caregiver burnout, caregivers need to take breaks and decompress.

Here are some tips that helped my husband, who was an excellent caregiver despite having his father and wife hospitalized at the same time, a demanding job, young kids, pets, and a household to manage.

Tips for Caregivers

* Keep up your physical health and strength. Try to get enough sleep and exercise and eat well. If you aren't taking care of yourself, how are you going to take care of your loved one?
* Continue doing the things that you enjoy. Running, blasting Stevie Ray Vaughan, and drinking beer in our dark basement gave my husband the opportunity to decompress and relax.
* Accept help. If you need to be at the hospital, ask for assistance with the pets, kids, and house. If you need to take a break, don't hesitate to reach out. People want to help you.
* Let it go. Your patient may make grumpy comments during her recovery. Don't take this personally. She will have a better attitude as her health improves. Invest in a good set of earbuds or turn up the stereo. Also, accept that the house and yard won't be perfect while you are busy caregiving. Focusing on your patient and maintaining your mental and physical health are the priorities.

Favorite Gifts Received: Ideas for Caregivers and Friends

My son and I loved receiving gifts during our recoveries. Our friends and family thought about our interests and tastes, and their presents buoyed our moods.

If your friends ask for suggestions, let them know whether you have any diet restrictions. Gifts of wine and beer can be enjoyed once you are off your pain medicines.

Recovery gift ideas:

* An orchid plant (this hardy flower blossomed for four months)
* Amazon gift cards or a Netflix subscription
* A soft blanket
* Magazines with lots of pictures and little substantive content
* Warm, fuzzy socks
* Movies and TV DVDs—comedies, action, mystery, and fantasy
* Edible fruit bouquet
* Loose-fitting PJs or a nightgown
* Meals or gift cards to local restaurants that deliver
* Invitation to have my family over for dinner while I rested
* Lunch of soup and a bagel or juices from a juice bar
* Books (a friend checked out her favorite books from the local library and dropped them off)
* A box of notecards and stamps
* Offers to clean my house, do my laundry, or put up my Christmas decorations
* Chocolate-covered strawberries and pound cake
* Blueberry muffins or banana bread
* Meditation CD or a meditation YouTube link
* Funny e-cards or links to videos (my brother sent hilarious YouTube videos via e-mail every other day)
* Texted photos from your high school or college days
* A warm latte
* An invitation to a party, a dinner, or something fun we can do together when I feel better

My eleven-year-old son, who had a challenging six-week summer surgery recovery period during which he was banned from swimming and wore an arm cast, loved the following gifts:

* Ice cream
* Books—anything by Rick Riordan or Brandon Mull, *The Kingdom Keepers* series, joke books, and sports books
* Links to fantasy baseball or football leagues so he could play with friends while lying on the couch
* Comic books
* Movies
* Cartoons
* Gift cards for the iPhone, iPad, Xbox Connect
* Video games like "Clash of Clans" or sports video games he could play remotely with friends
* Cookies, candy, and brownies
* Gift card to an ice cream store
* E-mails with links to funny YouTube videos

THANK-YOU TEXTS OR E-MAILS INSTEAD OF THANK-YOU NOTES

Handwritten notes that mention how grateful you are for the meals and gifts your friends provide are always appreciated. They are the gold standard of gratitude. But recovering from surgery (or serious illness or childbirth) can be fatiguing and disorienting. During these trying times, you might not have the energy to track down addresses, lick unsavory envelope glue, and hobble to the mailbox. If I had sent handwritten notes early in my recovery, I would not have had the stamina to make a grocery list or brush my teeth.

When I provide meals and gifts for sick friends, I appreciate their quick thank-you texts or e-mails. Thank-you texts give me a chance to check in on a recovering friend in real time and are a perfectly fine replacement for handwritten notes. If you receive a meal or gift through a delivery service, it's nice to let your friend know that you got it. I tried to text right after receiving a delivery so I wouldn't forget and my friend wouldn't wonder if her gift ever made it. My sister liked getting thank-you texts for the meals she sent and would text back asking which soup or salad we liked best.

Another possibility is to have your spouse, friend, or child draft the thank-you text or e-mail. They could also write or illustrate thank-you notes that you can sign. You or your partner could type a general letter of thanks and post it to your Facebook page or have your organizer send it out via e-mail. One of the best things you can do to thank your friends is to pay their kindness forward and help them or someone else during a challenging time.

CHAPTER 10

Resuming Your Life

WHEN YOU CAN SPEND AN entire day without thinking about your surgery, you have returned to normal. Rather than feeling achy, you are busy picking up the dry cleaning, unloading the dishwasher, and polishing off leftover pizza crusts while hunched over the sink.

Because you feel normal again, you might not want to spend time thinking about or discussing your health issues.

DISCUSSING YOUR HEALTH (OR NOT)

When someone asks, "How *are* you?" you can share as much or as little of your personal health information as you choose. You are not in front of Judge Judy, under oath, or wrapped in Wonder Woman's golden lasso. If asked specifically, "What is going on with your health?" you still have no obligation to share details of your recent blood transfusion or biopsy results. It's fine to ignore the question, change the topic, or be evasive.

During my recoveries, I didn't want to discuss my medical issues. Or be treated as Sickly Surgery Girl. So when a friend or

138

acquaintance asked me about my health, I would change the subject as soon as possible.

Friend or acquaintance: "How is your health? What is really going on with you?"

Me: "I'm getting a little better each day. I'm hoping to put the whole thing behind me. What are you up to?"

Me: "I'm doing as well as can be expected. But let's talk about something else. I have been meaning to ask you, which TV shows have you been enjoying lately? I need something good to watch."

If someone persists in making relentless inquiries about your health, you might be tempted to politely snap, "PLEASE MIND YOUR OWN DAMN BEESWAX!" and leave the room. But try to give people the benefit of the doubt. Who knows? They may have secretly scheduled the same surgery or have a relative who needs the same operation you had. Just explain that it's not fun for you to talk about your health. Then bring up the latest movies, political scandals, or *Saturday Night Live* skits.

The good news is that by five months after your surgery, everyone forgets about your operation and treats you like they always did.

DISGUISING YOUR SURGERY

If you don't want people to know that you had surgery, clothing and accessories can hide the aftermath of some operations. For a thyroid removal, a tummy tuck, or a breast reduction, scarves, vests, billowing shirts, and large necklaces can provide coverage and distraction. For plastic surgery, like an eyelid lift or nose job, you can change something else about your appearance before revealing your new look. For example, you could widen your lipstick lines or change your hair color. If someone comments that you look "different," you can attribute it to new red highlights or larger lip lines.

AVOIDING SURGERY COMPARISONS

Well-intentioned friends and acquaintances might compare other people's experiences with the surgery you had. In order to encourage you, they might say things like, "My cousin Jen played nine holes of golf four days after her robotic hysterectomy. She said the surgery was a breeze," or "Jen, that lady I work with, cut her lawn with a push mower five days after her abdominal surgery. Then she mulched."

Great for Jen! Four weeks after my hysterectomy, I buckled my seat belt unassisted. Good for me! Everyone recovers at a different rate; it's silly to compare yourself to others. Jen might have had a different type of hysterectomy, or she could be ten years younger than me. She might have had fewer complications or coexisting medical conditions. I could just be a slow healer, and Jen might possess super regenerating genes.

It's not productive to engage in the Keeping Up with the Jens of Recovery. As long as you follow your doctor's recovery timeline, you are on the right track. If you have any concerns about your progress, check in with your medical team. Ignore your friend's comments about Jen. Let her know that you are following your medical team's recovery advice.

RESUMING DRIVING

Before driving after major surgery, you need to be off all medications that could affect your judgment. You also should get your doctor's permission to drive. And it's a good idea to check that you are physically ready. Prior to heading out on the road, sit in a parked car and make sure you can comfortably stomp on the break, turn in your seat, and wear a seat belt. Start with short local trips, and take your time getting used to being back behind the wheel.

I resumed driving five weeks after major surgery by backing out of my driveway. Since I felt a weird pulling sensation and a little weakness, I stopped and decided to wait a few more days. I then went out for a Sunday-morning drive with my husband, who, to be honest, is not always confident in my driving skills even when I am 100 percent well. But my husband is a supportive spouse. He sat white-knuckled in the passenger seat as I hunched over the wheel like Rumpelstiltskin. While I drove fifteen miles an hour through our quiet neighborhood, he offered pointers, such as "A parked car is coming up on your right! It's thirty yards away! On your RIGHT!" and "There is a red stop sign ahead! RED MEANS STOP!" (Although I had been driving without incident for the last twenty-nine years, these reminders kept us safe.) I progressed from those neighborhood drives to successful trips to the grocery store and later branched out to highway driving.

GOING ON AN ERRAND BY YOURSELF

Like a teenager with a new license, you might be anxious to get out of the house for your first solo trip to a store. There are some things to keep in mind before going on your first errand:

- Plan your first outing to a small local store, such as a drugstore that you know well. Avoid the two-mile loop from the bananas to the Tylenol in Walmart.
- Plan to go in the morning, when you might have more energy and the stores are less crowded.
- Ask the store employees for help if you need assistance lifting heavy items into your cart or car.
- Use a motorized cart if needed.
- Let your kids or partner move the items from the car and put them away.

Soon you will be completing multiple errands in an outing. As you return to normal, you will think less about managing a trip to the supermarket and more about staying in for a romantic evening with your partner.

Sex after Surgery

Surgeons do not always specify when you can return to amorous activities. But if your doctor says no physical exertion for a month after surgery, that includes lifting, exercise, and sex. Your surgeon wants to make sure your incisions are healing and that you do not place too much stress on the stitches. The amount of time you need to take off from bouncing in the boudoir will depend on what type of surgery you had and how you are recovering.

After surgery, resuming your sex life might not be a pressing matter. You might be more focused on getting back to the office or weaning off pain medicine so you can enjoy a bottle of wine. Once you feel well enough to go back to work and maintain an exercise routine, you might want to resume intimacy. But check with your medical team to see if you are cleared for sex. Doctors get sex questions every day, and we really shouldn't feel embarrassed about bringing these things up. Your physician is a professional. He is there to help. He has been trained to control his demeanor and recognize body-part nicknames. (Your doctor won't collapse into a heap of giggles if you, like Ned Flanders, refer to your "dingly dangly diddly ding dong.")

Since I was raised to strictly use medically incorrect terms like "private lady parts" only when absolutely necessary and *never* in public, I wasn't entirely comfortable bringing up sex questions with my surgeon. But it was my job to talk openly to my doctor about my recovery. When I boldly whispered, "Is everything ready to go down there?" my surgeon, who could barely hear me, understood my pointing and hand gestures and had no problem addressing my question.

Besides thinking about sex as you return to normal, you might also want to focus on your bank account. A few days or weeks after surgery, your medical bills and explanation of benefits will arrive. The following section details how to check your bills for accuracy.

Review Your Medical Bills for Accuracy

Mistakes are often made during the complex medical billing process. It's worth taking the time to see if you have been overcharged. While doing the bills is boring, saving money by catching an error is not.

Before getting started, it's helpful to have a general understanding of the billing process. For someone who has health insurance, it usually works like this:

A doctor or nurse does a procedure, makes a diagnosis, or runs a test and bills your insurance company using specific codes for each procedure or test. Your insurance company gets the bill and checks to see if the coded items are covered. If they are covered, the company decides how much it will pay. The insurance company generates an explanation of benefits (EOB). The EOB describes the test or procedure, what the insurance company will cover, and what *you* will need to pay. The EOB is sent to you and your hospital and doctors. The EOB is *not* a bill, but a dark foreshadowing of your bill. The hospital (and doctors') billing staff will generate your actual bill based on the EOB. They will send the bill to you, and you will have a certain number of days to pay it.

In order to understand the different sections of your medical bill, check out the nonprofit FAIR Health website at Fairhealthconsumer. org. They have a helpful page called "How to Review Your Medical Bills," which is a source for the following information.

How to Review Your Medical Bills

Step one: Spread out the bills in front of you. Get a pencil and review the bills for accuracy. Circle anything questionable.

Check for the following:

* Have you been incorrectly charged for anything twice?
* Are there charges for a test that was canceled or a doctor you never saw?
* If you checked out of the hospital in the morning, were you charged for a full day by mistake?

* Is there an outrageously large charge?
* Do the numbers add up? If you have a 10 percent copay, make sure you are not charged more than that.
* Are there any uncoded items that were denied?
* Are there any items that your insurance company says are not covered but you think, after glancing at your policy, should be?
* Does the bill match the corresponding EOB?

<u>Step two</u>: Call your hospital or doctor's billing department and review any potential errors. The doctors and hospital want to be paid, so they might help you find codes or get procedures covered.

<u>Step three</u>: Pay your medical bills on time. Making late payments or skipping payments could affect your credit score, and your bill could be sent to a collection agency.

<u>Step four</u>: If you can't pay the bill on time, contact the billing office. They might agree to a reduction in the amount you owe, work with you on an extended payment schedule, or possibly offer you financial aid.

Besides thinking about money as you slowly return to normal, you might be contemplating cooking again. You may be missing the sound of bacon crackling in your skillet or the aroma of your homemade chicken chili. The following section can help you ease back into the kitchen.

COOKING AGAIN WITH DINNER ASSEMBLIES

Friends and family delivered delicious meals for the first five weeks after my surgeries. By week six, I was ready to resume my role as the family chef. The plan was to alternate among frozen meals, a cold cereal buffet, and dinner assemblies. Chopping, lifting heavy pots, and grating can be tiring after surgery.

Dinner assemblies are practical, everyday recipes based on precut, preshredded, prewashed, and jarred ingredients. They require a small amount of standing, stirring, and cleanup and are made with a limited number of ingredients that you assemble into a meal.

While everything, of course, does taste better when you cook from scratch, the idea here is to aim low. During my recoveries, I was just trying to get something warm and edible on the table so I could go back to bed. Once I felt completely well again, I could join the Slow Food movement.

Here's an overview of dinner-assembly ingredients that can be found at your local supermarket.

Ideal Ingredients	Dinner-Assembly Ingredients
Fresh carrots from the local farmers' market	Bag of baby carrots from Kroger's supermarket
Block of parmesan cheese that you hand grate	Plastic container of grated parmesan cheese
Homemade marinara sauce or salsa using tomatoes from your garden	Jar of tomato sauce or salsa from the grocery store
Head of lettuce and homemade dressing	Package of prewashed chopped salad that includes dressing and toppings

Your own homemade taco seasoning	Package of McCormick taco seasoning
Spices, meats, breadcrumbs, and eggs to make meatballs from scratch	Premade, uncooked meatballs from the meat counter at the grocery store
Homemade enchilada sauce	Pouch of Frontera enchilada sauce or bottle of Trader Joe's enchilada sauce
Chicken roasted in your oven	Rotisserie chicken from supermarket
Organic butter for greasing baking sheets	Cooking spray or baking sheet lined with foil or parchment paper for quick cleanup
Your own marinade for grass-fed pork loin or organic chicken breast	Preseasoned or marinated chicken breast or Hormel pork loin

The following dinner assemblies—it would be a stretch to call some of them recipes—are easy to make and difficult to ruin. They should feed a family of four.

Cooking premarinated meats, which roast while you rest, is a good place to start. If you still have lifting restrictions, your partner or an older kid can be your sous chef and move pans in and out of the oven for you.

PREMARINATED MEATS

Supermarkets sell premarinated meats that are prepared in house, such as the lemon-herb chicken breast and meat kabobs that I get at my local

Publix. They also have commercially produced products, like Hormel boneless pork loin, which comes in a variety of flavors. Prepare these by following the baking directions on the package. (If you don't have an instant-read meat thermometer, get one; it will make your life easier.) Pair the cooked meat with one of the side dishes below.

SIMPLE SIDES

During my recoveries, I served four categories of side dishes: salad from a bag, oven-roasted vegetables, vegetables steamed in the microwave, and couscous, which, unlike rice, is impossible for me to ruin. (One day, if my counter space miraculously grows, I will buy a rice cooker, which will solve all my rice issues.)

1) Salad from a bag. My family likes the prechopped Southwestern, Caesar, and Asian salads, which include dressings and toppings. My kids can assemble these.

2) Microwave vegetables. Put a precut vegetable of your choice, like broccoli or cauliflower, in a microwave-safe dish. Sprinkle with a small amount of water (about two tablespoons) and cover. Microwave for a minute and a half, check see how it looks, and continue to microwave it for another minute. (Microwaves vary in power, so these times are a guideline.) Add salt, butter, lemon pepper, or whatever else you like on your vegetables before serving.

3) Oven-roasted vegetables. Choose a pound to a pound and a half of a vegetable, such as baby potatoes, sweet potatoes, onions, asparagus, red or yellow pepper, carrots, squash, zucchini, or cauliflower. (Many of these can be found precut at the supermarket.) Line a baking pan with parchment paper or aluminum foil. Place the cut-up vegetables in a single layer on the pan. You want the vegetables to be approximately the same size so they cook evenly. Toss the vegetables on the pan with about two

tablespoons of olive oil, sprinkle with about a teaspoon of salt, and spread them out evenly. Bake in the oven at 400°F. Denser, larger vegetable chunks will take longer to cook. Vegetables like potatoes, carrots, squash, and onions take about thirty to forty minutes. Cauliflower, brussels sprouts, and broccoli roast in about twenty to twenty-five minutes, and asparagus, tomatoes, peppers, and zucchini take ten to twenty minutes to roast. Check the vegetables as you get close to the finishing time. Depending on your taste, you can season the vegetables with salt, pepper, garlic salt, or red pepper flakes (which are good on cauliflower) before or after cooking.

4) Boxed couscous or microwave rice. Follow the directions on the bag or box.

Easy Pork Tenderloin

The following marinade is simple to make and the tenderloin consistently turns out well.

Five-Ingredient Roast Pork Tenderloin

Ingredients:

* 2 pounds (approximately) boneless pork tenderloin
* ½ cup olive oil
* ½ cup balsamic vinegar, like Trader Joe's or Colavita
* 2 tablespoons steak seasoning, like McCormick Montreal steak seasoning or Borsari seasoning
* 3 garlic cloves, chopped
* Optional: precut carrots, sweet potatoes, butternut squash, and/or onions can be roasted under or alongside the pork tenderloin as it cooks.

Directions:

1. Stir the olive oil, balsamic vinegar, garlic, and steak seasoning together in a bowl for about 2 minutes until the steak
   seasoning dissolves.
2. Place the pork in a gallon-size ziplock bag and pour the marinade over it.
3. Marinate in the refrigerator for at least 3 hours to overnight.
4. Heat the oven to 400°F.
5. Place the vegetables (if using) and pork in a glass baking dish
   and cook for about 30–40 minutes until the internal temperature of the pork reaches 145°F. Let it sit for five minutes
   before slicing.

Note: This recipe was adapted from Allrecipes.com.

PACKAGED PASTA AND JARRED SAUCE ASSEMBLIES

If you have someone around who can lift a big pot of boiled pasta water
for you, then boxed penne with a jarred sauce such as marinara, meat,
vodka, or pesto is an option. To make things interesting, combine jarred
sauces: mix a cup of Newman's Own Alfredo with a jar of pesto sauce
if you prefer a creamy pesto. To increase the protein, toss in some microwaved sausage or meatballs (like Aidell's Italian-style links and meatballs) or add low-fat shredded mozzarella on top. A bagged Caesar salad
or microwaved broccoli could complete the meal.

If you don't want to deal with a heavy pot of boiling water, try a
baked pasta recipe. You can vary the type of tortellini (cheese, chick-
en, or mushroom) and sauces according to your taste.

Tortellini Bake
Ingredients:

* 1 pound refrigerated tortellini (such as Buitoni cheese or chicken tortellini)
* 2 cups vodka sauce (from a jar)
* 2 cups marinara sauce (from a jar)
* 3 cups prewashed baby spinach (or baby kale)
* 1 cup shredded mozzarella cheese

Directions:

1. Heat oven to 375°F.
2. Stir uncooked tortellini, spinach, and sauces in a bowl.
3. Pour into a greased 13" by 9" baking dish.
4. Top with the shredded cheese. Cover and bake for about 20 minutes. If feeling motivated, uncover and bake for 5 more minutes until cheese is bubbly.

Note: We like our pasta extra saucy. You can adjust the amount and type of sauce to your preferences. This recipe was adapted from the ThisGalCooks.com.

Ravioli Acting as Lasagna
Ingredients:

* 1 jar (25–28 oz.) marinara sauce or marinara with meat sauce
* 1 package (25–28 oz.) refrigerated cheese (or chicken or mushroom) ravioli

- 1 ½ cups grated mozzarella cheese
- ½ cup grated parmesan cheese
- 3 cups prewashed baby spinach (or baby kale)

Directions:

1. Heat oven to 375°F.
2. Spread ¾ of a cup of the marinara sauce on the bottom of the prepared baking dish.
3. Place half of the ravioli in a single layer over sauce.
4. Put on a layer of spinach and top with half of each kind of cheese.
5. Put on another layer of ravioli and remaining sauce and cheese.
6. Cover with aluminum foil and bake approximately 20 minutes. Uncover and bake for 5 minutes more so cheese is fully melted.

Note: Variations on this recipe could be butternut-squash ravioli with a jar of Newman's Own Alfredo sauce or a package of lobster ravioli with a jar of vodka sauce. This recipe was adapted from RealSimple.com.

Meatball Sandwiches
Ingredients:

- 1 pound uncooked premade meatballs from meat counter of grocery store (do not use frozen meatballs)
- 1 jar of your favorite marinara sauce
- 6 hamburger rolls
- 1 cup shredded mozzarella cheese

Directions:

1. Cook meatballs in marinara sauce on low for about 25 minutes until they reach an internal temperature of 145°F.
2. Place them on hamburger rolls; top with shredded mozzarella. (If you have extra sauce left over, you can refrigerate or freeze it and use it on pasta.)

ROTISSERIE CHICKEN ASSEMBLIES

Rotisserie chickens are convenient, versatile, affordable, chock-full of protein, and something my whole family will eat. I try to purchase rotisserie chickens no more than two hours before dinner so I can serve one that night. I keep one chicken in its original container, in one of those shiny silver bags that keep cold foods cold and hot foods hot. If I buy rotisserie chicken three hours before dinner, I put it and its juices into a Pyrex dish, cover it with foil, and keep it warm in an oven at two hundred degrees Fahrenheit. (This is what the Publix rotisserie-chicken guy suggested, and it's worked for us.)

I usually buy two rotisserie chickens at a time, one to keep warm for dinner and one to shred for quesadillas or enchiladas later in the week. It's easier to shred the chicken when it's still warm, and the meat can be used in soup, chili, wraps, and casseroles.

ROTISSERIE CHICKEN AND CUMIN CARROTS
Ingredients:

* 1 rotisserie chicken still warm from supermarket
* 1 package baby carrots

- 2 tablespoons olive oil
- ½ teaspoon salt
- 1 ½ teaspoons cumin powder (or cumin seeds)

Directions:

1. Place the baby carrots on a baking sheet and mix them with the salt, olive oil, and cumin.
2. Bake the cumin carrots at 400°F for about 30 minutes.
3. Serve the carrots with the warm rotisserie chicken.

Note: You can substitute sweet potatoes for the carrots. This cumin carrots recipe was adapted from Epicurious.com.

CHEESE AND CHICKEN QUESADILLAS

Ingredients:

- 8 8" flour tortillas
- 2 cups shredded rotisserie chicken
- 2 cups shredded Mexican-style cheese
- 1 jar of your favorite salsa
- Optional: avocado

Directions:

1. Spray a baking pan with nonstick spray.
2. Place the tortillas on the pan and evenly divide the shredded rotisserie chicken and shredded cheese among the tortillas. (You can add a tablespoon of salsa and a slice of avocado to the cheese and chicken filling for additional flavor.)

3. Fold the flour tortilla in half; spray with nonstick spray.
4. Bake on a cookie sheet at 375°F for about 8–10 minutes, until golden brown.
5. Serve with salsa.

Note: These can be made ahead in the morning. Keep them in the refrigerator until you are ready to eat, and then stick them in the oven.

<u>Chopped Chicken Salad</u>: Add about 2 cups of shredded rotisserie chicken to bagged chopped Caesar, Southwest, or Asian salad.

CHICKEN ENCHILADAS
Ingredients:

* 8 8" flour tortillas
* 3 cups shredded rotisserie chicken (I usually get roughly 3 cups of shredded chicken from a 2-pound bird.)
* Bottle, pouch, or can of enchilada sauce, such as Frontera red chili enchilada sauce or green chili enchilada sauce, Trader Joe's enchilada sauce, 365 brand, or Las Palmas green chile enchilada sauce
* 2 cups shredded Monterey Jack cheese from a bag
* 1 jar of your favorite salsa

Directions:

1. In a medium-size bowl, combine chicken, 1 cup salsa, and 1 cup cheese. Mix well to combine.
2. Put ⅓ cup enchilada sauce on the bottom of a prepared 9" by 13" baking dish.

3. Spoon about 3 tablespoons of the chicken mixture into the center of each tortilla, then roll them up and place seam-side down in the baking dish.
4. Pour the remaining enchilada sauce over the rolled-up tortillas.
5. Sprinkle cheese evenly on top.
6. Cover with foil and bake at 350°F for about 30 minutes.

Note: This recipe was adapted from Allrecipes.com. If we have extra taco meat from Taco Tuesdays, I use that as filling instead of the rotisserie chicken. If you want to eat these enchiladas at a later date, freeze them without the sauce or cheese topping, or they will get mushy. Add the sauce and sprinkle the shredded cheese right before you cover them with foil and bake at 350°F for about 50 minutes.

ONE-SHEET-PAN DINNERS

Baking your entire dinner on one sheet pan in the oven makes for an easy cleanup, especially if you line the baking sheet with a layer of foil or parchment paper. You can assemble a one-sheet-pan dinner in the morning and keep it in the fridge until you are ready for dinner.

ONE-PAN ZESTY ITALIAN CHICKEN AND POTATOES
Ingredients:

* 1 pound skinless chicken breasts or thighs
* 1 pound baby potatoes cut in half or precut sweet potatoes
* 4 tablespoons olive oil
* 1 Zesty Italian dressing packet (0.6 oz.)
* Salt and pepper

Directions:

1. Preheat oven to 400°F. Line a sheet pan with foil.
2. On the sheet pan, mix the potatoes with about 2 tablespoons olive oil, and lightly salt and pepper.
3. Place chicken on potatoes. Rub chicken with about 2 tablespoons olive oil, then salt and pepper.
4. Sprinkle the Italian seasoning packet evenly over the chicken and potatoes that are sticking out from under the chicken.
5. Bake, uncovered, for about 30–40 minutes, until chicken is done and potatoes are soft. Cooking time will depend on the thickness of the chicken.

Note: This recipe was adapted from Allrecipes.com.

CHICKEN FAJITAS BAKED ON A PAN

Ingredients:

*   1 pound (approximately) package of precut fajita vegetables. They can be labeled as fajita toppings or roast, steak, and pizza toppings, and include sliced onions, peppers, and mushrooms. If you can't find precut fajita vegetable packages, then slice 1 onion and 2 bell peppers ¼ inch thick.
*   1 pound skinless, boneless chicken breasts cut into ¼ inch slices (the meat department can slice them for you if you ask)
*   2 tablespoons olive oil
*   1 package fajita seasoning, such as McCormick
*   8 8"flour tortillas
*   Optional toppings: shredded Mexican-style cheese, prepared guacamole, sour cream, and salsa

Directions:

1. Preheat oven to 400°F.
2. Line a baking sheet with aluminum foil.
3. Place the chicken and vegetables on the baking sheet. Drizzle with the oil and fajita seasoning and toss to combine. Spread in an even layer.
4. Roast for about 30 minutes until the vegetables are tender and the chicken is cooked.
5. Serve with the tortillas and optional toppings.

ONE-PAN LEMON CHICKEN AND POTATOES

Ingredients:

* 1 pound chicken breasts or thighs
* 1/3 cup olive oil
* 1 pound baby potatoes, halved
* Juice of 1 lemon
* 2 tablespoons dried basil
* 2 tablespoons dried oregano
* 2 tablespoons lemon-pepper seasoning (like McCormick)
* 1 teaspoon salt

Directions:

1. Preheat oven to 400°F. Line a large sheet pan with foil.
2. Combine olive oil, lemon juice, basil, lemon pepper, oregano, and salt in a bowl.

3. Place chicken and potatoes on the sheet pan. Drizzle with olive oil mixture and toss to combine.
4. Bake, uncovered, for about 30–40 minutes, until chicken is no longer pink and reaches an internal temperature of 165°F and potatoes are done.

Note: This recipe was adapted from Greek Lemon Chicken and Potato bake at Allrecipes.com.

Taco Meat Recipes

Tacos are popular in my house because everyone can choose their own toppings. I make two pounds of taco meat on Taco Tuesdays, one pound for tacos and one pound for either enchilada filling or the Taco Twist Pasta.

Tacos
Ingredients:

* 8 taco shells (we prefer 8"flour tortillas)
* 1 pound ground beef (or ground turkey)
* 1 package McCormick taco seasoning
* 1 jar of your favorite salsa
* Optional ingredients for taco toppings: avocado, shredded Mexican-style cheese, prewashed lettuce, premade guacamole, and whatever else you like in your tacos.

Directions:

1. Brown taco meat per the directions on the McCormick taco seasoning packet. (I usually use about ¾ packet for a pound of meat.)
2. Add about ¾ cup salsa to the taco meat mixture.
3. Spoon prepared taco meat into flour or corn taco shells.
4. Serve with desired toppings.

TACO TWIST PASTA

Note: This recipe does require boiling spiral pasta.

Ingredients:
* 1 pound cooked and prepared taco meat, as above
* 24–26 oz. jar marinara sauce
* 1 cup jarred salsa
* 1 package spiral pasta
* 1 cup sour cream
* 1 cup shredded Mexican-style cheese

Directions:

1. Cook spiral pasta until al dente per package directions and set aside.
2. In a large saucepan, mix salsa, cooked and seasoned taco meat, marinara sauce, ½ cup shredded cheese, and sour cream. Stir and bring to a low boil, cooking for about 5 minutes.
3. Combine the cooked but still warm pasta with sauce and spread it in a 9" by 13" pan.

4. Sprinkle ½ cup shredded Mexican cheese on top of pasta.
5. Cover with aluminum foil and bake for about 20 minutes at 375°F.

Note: This recipe was adapted from Tasteofhome.com.

Frozen Shrimp Recipes

Shrimp is high in protein and cooks in about three minutes. Deveined and shelled frozen shrimp is easy to use and keep on hand. I buy it in a bag at my local grocery store.

Quick Spicy Shrimp over Couscous

Ingredients:

* 2 tablespoons olive oil
* 4 garlic cloves, minced
* Juice of 1 lemon
* ½ teaspoon crushed red pepper flakes
* 24 frozen, uncooked shrimp, peeled and deveined
* 2 teaspoons steak seasoning blend, like McCormick Montreal seasoning or Borsari seasoning
* Box of couscous (Start couscous before cooking shrimp)

Directions:

1. Heat a large skillet over medium-high heat.
2. Add olive oil, then garlic, red pepper flakes, steak seasoning blend, and shrimp.

3. Cook shrimp for 3–4 minutes or until just pink.
4. Serve over couscous.

Note: This recipe was adapted from Rachael Ray.

Panda Express–like Sweet Fire Shrimp
Ingredients:

* 24 frozen, uncooked shrimp, shelled and deveined
* 1 tablespoon olive oil
* 1 red bell pepper, chopped
* 1 to 1 ½ cups diced pineapple, fresh or canned, drained
* ½ cup Thai sweet chili sauce, or more, to taste (you can buy this pink sauce at your grocery store)
* Optional: Rice or couscous to go with the shrimp

Directions:

1. Heat olive oil in a large skillet over medium-high heat, add shrimp, and cook about 2 minutes until just pink.
2. Add bell pepper and pineapple and cook until tender, about 2–4 minutes.
3. Stir in Thai sweet chili sauce until combined.
4. Serve while hot.

Note: You can substitute cooked chicken nuggets for the shrimp if you don't have shrimp on hand. This recipe was adapted from Damndelicioucous.com.

SLOW COOKER RECIPES

A slow cooker, or a Crock-Pot, allows you to throw ingredients together and walk away from the kitchen for hours as your dinner simmers and develops. No standing, stirring, or peering under the lid is necessary.

You can freeze the ingredients of Crock-Pot meals together in plastic ziplock bags before your surgery. There are several websites dedicated to Crock-Pot freezer-meal recipes.

Keep in mind that if you have lifting restrictions, you should have someone place the slow cooker on the counter for you.

CROCK-POT BARBEQUE SHREDDED CHICKEN SANDWICH

Ingredients:

* 1–2 pounds skinless, boneless chicken breasts
* 1 bottle good barbecue sauce, like Famous Dave's or Sweet Baby Ray's
* 1 shallot or onion, chopped
* 1 package hamburger buns
* Premade coleslaw for topping

Directions:

1. Put in a slow cooker liner or spray pot with nonstick spray.
2. Put chopped onion on the bottom of the slow cooker.
3. Place chicken breasts on top of the onions and pour the barbecue sauce evenly over chicken. Cover all the chicken with the barbecue sauce (you might not use the whole jar).

4. Cover and cook on low for about 6–7 hours. After about 5 hours, shred the chicken using a knife and fork and let it soak up the sauce.
5. Put chicken on buns. Top with coleslaw and, if desired, more barbecue sauce.

Note: This recipe was adapted from Food.com.

Stovetop or Slow Cooker White Chicken Chili
Ingredients:

* 6 cups chicken broth
* 3 cups shredded rotisserie chicken (or see slow cooker method below, which uses uncooked chicken breasts)
* 2 15 oz. cans white cannellini beans, drained
* 2 cups premade salsa verde (this green salsa can be found next to the red ones)
* 2 teaspoons ground cumin
* ½ teaspoon chili powder
* Optional toppings: shredded cheese, crumbled tortilla chips, avocado, Fritos, goldfish crackers

Directions:

Stovetop method:

1. Put chicken broth, shredded rotisserie chicken, beans, green salsa, chili powder, and cumin in a medium saucepan and stir to combine.

2. Heat over medium-high heat until boiling, then cover and reduce heat to medium-low and simmer for at least 10 minutes.
3. Season to taste; if needed, add more chili powder and salt.
4. Serve warm with toppings.

Slow cooker method:

1. Use a slow cooker liner or spray pot with nonstick spray.
2. Add chicken broth, 2 uncooked boneless, skinless chicken breasts, beans, salsa, chili powder, and cumin to slow cooker and stir to combine.
3. Cook on low for 6–8 hours.
4. Shred the chicken. Season to taste; if needed, add more chili powder and salt.
5. Serve warm with desired toppings.

Note: This recipe was adapted from Gimmesomeoven.com.

KEEPING YOUR SURGERY RESOLUTIONS
Unlike the traditional New Year's weight-loss resolution, which is usually broken on January 8 in a Burger King booth, surgery resolutions can last a lifetime. Surgery is expensive, anxiety-provoking, and uncomfortable. No one wants to have to repeat it.

Patients often make health resolutions after an operation. You might vow to exercise five times a week after your quadruple heart bypass. Or you might commit to eating a high-fiber diet after colon surgery. Perhaps you promise to maintain a healthy weight so you don't put too much pressure on your artificial knee and cause it to deteriorate.

A major operation can give us a sense of our mortality, which is a strong motivator. Bill Clinton traded in jalapeño cheeseburgers for textured vegetable protein patties after heart surgery and explained, "I wanted to live to be a grandfather." So he made a permanent resolution to eat a healthier diet. Seven years and hundreds of bean burgers later, he achieved his goal and enjoys two adorable grandchildren.

After my last surgery, I was told to cut way back on the booze and to exercise for forty-five minutes a day while doing an activity that "puts a smile on my face." I was not thrilled with this advice. Who has the time and inclination to exercise forty-five minutes *every day* (and beam about it)? And abandon beer? Beer has made my life better in many, many ways—from improving the taste of my tacos to mitigating the awkwardness of my first date with my husband.

But ultimately I want to stay in good health for my family and myself, so I try to carry out these resolutions. If I look at my overall behavior for the last two years, I have been moderately successful. That's because when I break my surgery resolutions, which happens about every other month, I jump right back on the resolution bandwagon.

The following are tips that help me.

Maintaining Surgery Resolutions
Step one: Make the surgery resolution meaningful to you. Then break its execution into concrete baby steps. Frame the

resolution so that it matters. Instead of saying you need to lower your cholesterol, lose weight, or become a teetotaler, try these:

Resolution: I need to reduce my cholesterol so I can avoid another heart surgery. I want to be in good health to take my niece on a trip to New York City for her eighteenth birthday.

Specific baby step: I am going to exchange my daily Egg McMuffin for a sourdough or whole-grain English muffin.

Resolution: I need to lose weight so my knee replacement doesn't wear down. I want to stay in shape to continue building houses with Habitat for Humanity.

Specific baby step: I will walk around my neighborhood for half an hour after work.

Resolution: I need to cut back on the booze after my liver operation. I don't want to go back under the knife or have to find a new liver.

Specific baby steps: I will meet friends for lunch or brunch, meals when people are less likely to drink. I will cut back from three glass of wine a night to one glass. I will drink only on Saturdays.

Step two: Link your surgery resolution to something or someone you enjoy. By associating your resolution with something positive, you are more apt to complete it.

Ideas:

* Treat yourself to a smoothie after your exercise class. Run or walk to a coffee shop for your morning caffeine fix.
* Watch your favorite TV show only when you are on the treadmill or exercise bike.
* Make it social: set up walking, hiking, dancing, tennis, golf, yoga, or aerobics class outings with friends or family. Local YMCAs and Meetup.com have exercise, running, and walking groups.

Step three: Make easy substitutions. Make the least painful healthy replacements first.

Ideas:

* Switch to low-fat dairy products or low-calorie drinks that taste like the original.
* Walk up to the Starbucks counter rather than sitting in the drive-through line. Have stevia instead of sugar in your latte.
* Order a low-alcohol beer instead of a high-gravity one, or ask for only a splash of vodka in your drink.

Step four: Be flexible about how you get your exercise. When it comes to exercise, every little bit helps. Leave a pair of sneakers in the car or in your office so you can sneak in last-minute walks wherever and whenever.

Ideas:

* Leave the office (or your house or apartment) and walk to get coffee. Walk to a restaurant for lunch. Walk or bike as part of your commute.

- Pace while talking on the phone. While you are in the house, pace if you are texting or surfing the Internet on your phone.
- Take a lap around the inside of the mall before and after going to a store. Do a lap around the inside of the supermarket with your cart before checking out.
- If you are ten minutes early to a meeting or activity, do a quick stroll. Walk during your kid's soccer, lacrosse, or baseball practice.

Step five: Get back on track fast. Everyone breaks their health resolutions. It's inevitable. We get a bad head cold and stay curled up in bed. A work deadline keeps us holed up in the office. We go on vacation and end up on a piña colada crawl. When this happens, stay calm. It's expected and inevitable, and part of maintaining surgery health resolutions. The following tips can help you get back on track:

<u>Don't abandon a resolution because of a slipup.</u> Eating a sleeve of Thin Mints Girl Scout cookies is not a legitimate reason to ditch your entire diet. A couple of hours of exercise can make up for the slipup.

<u>Understand what caused the slipup and adapt.</u> If you are no longer showing up at your exercise class or your group run, why isn't it working for you? Is the run too early in the morning? Does the exercise class conflict with something else you'd rather do? Is the instructor boring? Adapt—change teachers, classes, or activities. Notice patterns: Are you hungover on Friday mornings? Have you thought about changing your Thursday-night activities?

<u>Get back on track.</u> Don't wait for a Monday, January 1, or the next full moon to restart your resolution. Resume it today. If needed, bribe or reward yourself to get going.

If falling down and breaking our resolutions is bound to happen, it can be just as inevitable that we get up and keep moving forward.

◆ ◆ ◆

Hopitalese Simplified: A Guide to Medical Jargon

On occasion, I use medical words that don't mean what I think they mean. And I often mispronounce them. For example, I asked if the "fascist" in my stomach had healed when I should have used the word "fascia." (Fascia means connective tissue.) My mispronunciation confused my nurse. Did her patient think she had a mini-Mussolini living in her tummy?

In order to clarify my medical questions, I looked up medical jargon, also known as "hospitalese," on the Cleveland Clinic website, Johns Hopkins Health Library web page, and MedlinePlus.gov. I used these sources for most of the definitions below, which I tried to translate into regular English.

Adhesion: Internal scar tissue that can stick organs together, which might need to be unstuck with surgery. We want to avoid these.

Advance directive or living will: These legal documents describe your medical care preferences if you are unable to make decisions for yourself. For more information, the Mayo Clinic website has a good overview of living wills.

Advocate: The person who goes to the hospital with you to be your supporter and champion throughout your stay.

Ambulant/ambulation: Able to walk; walking.

Anesthesia: Medication that relieves pain and sensation during surgery. It can be given via a breathing mask or a tube in your arm.

Anemia: A condition of not having enough healthy red blood cells. It can make you feel tired.

Antibiotic: A medicine that kills bacteria.

Anesthesiologist: A doctor who administers pain-relieving drugs during surgery.

Attending MD: A doctor with primary responsibility for patients in the hospital.

Autologous blood donation: The process of donating blood to yourself before surgery.

Benign: Not dangerous, not cancerous.

Blood pressure: A measure of how well blood circulates through your arteries. It is measured using a cuff that inflates and squeezes your arm.

Breathing tube: A tube that is inserted into your mouth and down your windpipe to ensure that you get enough oxygen and your lungs are protected when you're asleep and relaxed under general anesthesia. The tube is usually removed before you wake up.

Cardiologist: A doctor who specializes in heart disorders and heart disease.

Cellulitis: A deep infection of the skin caused by bacteria.

Chronic: Ongoing. A chronic illness is one that can continue for years.

Coagulate: To thicken or clot, used in reference to blood.

Contusion: A bruise.

Day surgery: A procedure that is performed when the patient leaves the same day. Also known as outpatient surgery.

Discharge: The point at which the patient leaves the hospital.

Drains: Used to direct fluid away from incisions after some surgeries, usually inserted under the incision to help speed healing and reduce infection.

Dressing: Gauze that goes under a bandage over an incision.

Deep vein thrombosis (DVT): A blood clot in a large vein.

External stitches: Stitches that you can see.

Electrocardiogram (EKG): A test that uses sound waves to examine the heart.

Electronic health record (EHR): A digital collection of all your health history, including allergies, medications, lab tests, and notes from the doctors you have seen.

Family and Medical Leave Act (FMLA): Legislation that allows eligible employees to take unpaid, job-protected leave for specific medical reasons.

Fascia: Connective tissue.

Fracture: Broken bone.

Hemorrhage: Bleeding.

Hematoma: Clotted blood that collects under the skin.

Hysterectomy: An operation to remove a woman's uterus.

Intensive care unit (ICU): An area in the hospital where seriously sick patients are cared for by specially trained nurses and doctors.

Incentive spirometer: A handheld device to keep your lungs healthy after surgery. It encourages you to take deep breaths.

Incision: A cut through the skin that is made during an operation. Also called a surgical wound.

Inpatient surgery: Surgery that requires the patient to spend the night in the hospital.

Internal stitches: Stitches that you cannot see because they are inside you.

Intubation/intubated: Having a breathing tube placed into the windpipe through the nose or mouth (see "breathing tube.")

Intravenous (IV) line: Also called a "drip." A small, flexible tube that is inserted into a vein to deliver fluid or medications.

Laparoscopy: A type of surgery done through one or more small incisions.

Medical imaging: Department where you can get an x-ray, MRI, or CT scan.

* <u>X-ray</u>: Small amounts of radiation form an image of your bones and organs.
* <u>Computed tomography (CT or CAT) scan</u>: Special x-rays and computer enhancement create more detailed three-dimensional images of body parts.
* <u>Ultrasound</u>: An ultrasound study uses sound waves to produce images of internal organs like kidneys or ovaries.
* <u>Magnetic resonance imaging (MRI)</u>: MRI uses magnets and radio waves to produce clear, detailed images of body organs, including the brain.

Minimally invasive surgery: When doctors use techniques like small incisions to operate. In general, minimally invasive surgery is associated with less pain and a shorter hospital stay than open surgery.

Nausea: Feeling sick to your stomach, as if you are going to vomit.

<u>Nonsteroidal anti-inflammatory drug (NSAID)</u>: Aspirin, Motrin, and Advil are examples of NSAIDs that you can buy over-the-counter, at a drugstore or supermarket, without a prescription. NSAIDs can help reduce pain or fever.

<u>Outpatient surgery</u>: The patient leaves the hospital, clinic, or doctor's office after surgery and doesn't spend the night.

<u>Patient-controlled analgesia (PCA)</u>: A computerized pump attached to an IV that allows patients to give themselves pain medicine (like morphine) by pressing a button.

<u>Phlebotomist</u>: A person who draws your blood or puts in an IV.

<u>Physician</u>: A medical doctor.

<u>Pneumonia</u>: Infection of the lungs

<u>Pulse / heart rate</u>: The number of times the heart beats in one minute.

<u>Pulse oximeter</u>: Monitors the saturation of oxygen in the blood. It looks like a fat clothespin and gently clips onto your finger.

<u>Radiology</u>: Department where x-rays and other imaging are done.

<u>Range of motion (ROM)</u>: How far a joint, like a knee or an elbow, can flex and extend.

<u>Residents</u>: Doctors in training. They have finished medical school.

Rhinorrhea: A runny nose.

Rounding: When doctors visit their hospitalized patients.

Scopolamine patch: A patch to wear behind the ear to prevent nausea. Often given before surgery (or on cruises to prevent seasickness).

Sequential compression device (SCD): A device to prevent blood clots by wrapping around your legs and inflating and deflating in intervals.

Sleep apnea: A sleeping disorder where you repeatedly stop and start breathing. If you think you have it, be sure to tell your doctor before surgery.

Sutures: Stitches.

Tachycardia: Fast heart rate (greater than one hundred beats per minute).

Transient ischemic attack (TIA): A mini-stroke. (A stroke happens when blood flow to an area of the brain is cut off.)

Topical: On the skin.

Urethra: Narrow channel through which urine passes from the bladder out of the body.

Urinalysis: Examination of a urine (pee) sample. A urinalysis can detect things like a urinary tract infection, kidney disease, and diabetes.

Urinary (Foley) catheter: A thin rubber tube that removes urine (pee) from the bladder.

Teaching hospital: Trains doctors and often is involved in research.

Vital signs: Measurements of four of the body's basic functions: temperature, blood pressure, respiration rate (breathing rate), and pulse (heart rate).

White blood cells: Disease-fighting cells in blood.

People You Might Meet in the Hospital

Doctors

Anesthesiologist: The anesthesiologist is the doctor who gives you inhaled gasses and drugs that keep you asleep and pain-free during surgery.

Attending physician: The attending physician is the doctor who is ultimately responsible for you during your hospital stay. If you are having surgery, it's usually your surgeon.

Hospitalist: Hospitalists are usually internal medicine doctors who only see hospitalized patients. (They don't have office hours.) There is often a team of them available twenty-four hours a day, and they know the hospital policies and doctors well.

Referring physician: The referring physician is the doctor who made the suggestion that you have surgery.

Primary-care physician: Your regular doctor. The doctor you see for checkups, routine screenings, and nonemergencies like sore throats. (Internists, family-practice doctors, and general practitioners are all considered primary-care physicians.) If you have an HMO, the primary-care doctor refers you to specialist doctors, including surgeons.

Specialists: Doctors who are experts in a particular field or body part. For example, a cardiologist is a heart specialist, a pulmonologist is a lung doctor, and a neurologist treats brain, spinal cord, and nerve disorders such as strokes, headaches, or multiple sclerosis.

<u>Surgeon</u>: A surgeon is a doctor who performs operations. There are general surgeons who perform operations like hernia repairs and appendectomies. There are also surgeons who specialize in operating on organs like the heart or brain.

<u>Fellows, residents, and interns</u>: These are physicians in the process of completing their medical training. You will find these individuals at teaching hospitals, where doctors are learning skills. Attending doctors teach the fellows, who then help teach the residents and interns.

NURSES

There are nurses everywhere you look in the hospital. There are pre-op nurses, post-op nurses, preadmitting nurses, and nurse anesthesiologists, among others. In the hospital, the nurses usually do not report to doctors but to nurse managers.

<u>Registered nurse (RN)</u>: An RN gives you medicines, checks your vitals, helps with bathing, and is in charge of the nurse assistants.

<u>Nurse assistants and nurse technicians</u>: These people help the registered nurses, but they usually can't give pain medicines.

<u>Nurse practitioner</u>: A nurse practitioner can do some tasks performed by doctors. After my son's elbow surgery, all of his follow-up appointments were with a nurse practitioner; we never saw the surgeon again.

<u>Nurse anesthetist (CRNA)</u>: A nurse who gives you anesthesia and is under the supervision of an anesthesiologist.

THERAPISTS

Physical therapist: A physical therapist helps patients move their bodies and get stronger. A physical therapist can help you walk again after hip surgery.

Occupational therapist: An occupational therapist can help you accomplish things you need to do in everyday life like grooming, bathing, and holding a fork.

Respiratory therapist: A respiratory therapist is a person who helps patients who need breathing treatments or oxygen.

OTHER IMPORTANT PLAYERS

Pharmacists: Hospitals have pharmacies on their premises. Pharmacists distribute a wide variety of medicines that are ordered by doctors for their patients. They often review the medicines for interactions and dosing accuracy.

Phlebotomist: A phlebotomist takes your blood or can help get an IV started.

Social workers: Social workers can help you plan for discharge from the hospital. They can arrange home-care visits from nurses or help you get into a rehabilitation or skilled nursing facility.

Technologists and technicians: These are the people who take x-rays and perform other procedures like drawing blood.

Housekeeping aide: A housekeeping aide is a person who cleans hospital rooms.

<u>Dietitian/nutritionist</u>: An expert in the area of nutrition and food who can give you advice on the best diet for your recovery.

<u>Chaplain</u>: Provides spiritual support to patients, their families, and medical staff.

Health Overview Sheet

- ☐ List any current health conditions (like diabetes, high blood pressure, etc.).
- ☐ List current medicines, including over-the-counter drugs, vitamins, and supplements.
- ☐ List how much you are taking. Also, note any medicines that you recently stopped taking.
- ☐ List any allergies to medicines, food, testing dyes, etc.
- ☐ List past operations and reactions to anesthesia or complications.
- ☐ List diseases or conditions in your immediate family (parents, siblings, and children).

Recovery Coverage Checklist

What Needs to Be Covered	Specific Action
Caring for the kids and pets while I'm in the hospital	
Shopping for groceries	
Preparing meals	
Getting a ride to post-op doctor's appointment	
Picking up prescriptions from pharmacy	
Paying bills	
Doing laundry	
Running dishwasher and putting dishes away	
Managing work	
Vacuuming and cleaning house	
Feeding and walking dog	
Getting kids to their activities and friends' birthday parties	
Hiring a neighborhood middle schooler to help with kids and dogs while I am home recovering	
Getting teeth cleaned at the dentist's office	
Volunteering	
Doing yard work	

Medicine Review at Discharge Chart

1. Review with your nurse your new prescriptions and how they work and document them.
2. Review the over-the-counter medicines that you can take during your recovery, such as Tylenol, Advil, heartburn medicines, and Miralax.
3. Review with your nurse the medications you were on before admission to the hospital and if they interact with your new prescriptions.
4. Review when you can resume taking your vitamins and supplements and if they interact with your prescribed drugs.

Medication Chart

Drug name (brand and generic)	What does this drug do? Why Am I taking it?	Dose and color of pill	When to take it/with or without food?	Date/Time Taken

Resources

Medical Websites

I found the following websites to have up-to-date medical information.

- MedlinePlus (www.medlineplus.gov), the National Institutes of Health website for patients and families
- Mayo Clinic (www.mayoclinic.org)
- University of California, San Francisco, Medical Center (www.ucsfhealth.org)
- Cleveland Clinic (www.clevelandclinic.org)
- Johns Hopkins Health Library (http://www.hopkinsmedicine.org/healthlibrary)
- Hospital for Special Surgery (www.hss.edu)

Hospital Rating Websites

You can check hospital ratings for things like patient safety and other patient experiences on the following sites:

- *US News and World Report*'s health section lists hospitals by specialty. http://health.usnews.com/best-hospitals/rankings
- Medicare.gov/HospitalCompare
- ConsumerReports.org/Health has a section that rates hospitals by state.

Caregiving and Meal-Planning Websites

These websites are free and make organizing offers of help easy. Friends can sign up to help by clicking on a link to a group calendar.

- Lotsa Helping Hands (lotsahelpinghands.com) organizes meal planning, childcare, rides, yard work, or anything else needed.
- Take Them a Meal (takethemameal.com) is also easy to use and focuses on providing meals.
- Meal Train (mealtrain.com) is specifically designed for organizing meals.

MEDICINE REMINDER PHONE APP

Medisafe is a free phone app that sends audible reminders to take your pain medicine and tracks when you last took it. See medisafe.com.

MEDICAL BILL OVERVIEW

In order to understand the different sections of your medical bill, check out the nonprofit FAIR Health website at Fairhealthconsumer.org. They have a helpful page called "How to Review Your Medical Bills."

CROWDFUNDING WEBSITES

If you or a loved one needs to raise money for medical bills and expenses, you could start a fund-raiser via the Internet on one of the following websites:

- Gofundme.com
- Giveforward.com
- Youcaring.com

Notes

Introduction

1. American Society of Anesthesiologists. "Patients Benefit from Enhanced Recovery Programs: Are Better Prepared for Surgery, Have Less Pain, Studies Show." Accessed January 9, 2017. https://www.asahq.org/about-asa/newsroom/news-releases/2016/10/patients-benefit-from-enhanced-recovery-programs.

Chapter 1

1. American Board of Family Medicine. "What Does Board-Certified Mean?" American Board of Family Medicine website. Accessed January 9, 2017. https://www.theabfm.org/diplomate/certified.aspx.
2. Mayo Clinic. "Minimally Invasive Surgery." Accessed January 12, 2017. http://www.mayoclinic.org/tests-procedures/minimally-invasive-surgery/home/ovc-20256733.

Chapter 2

1. "How to Find the Right Surgeon." *Consumer Reports*. Accessed January 9, 2017. http://www.consumerreports.org/cro/2012/04/how-to-find-the-right-surgeon/index.htm.
2. Amy Sarah Marshall, "Why Would I Want to Go to [a] Teaching Hospital? AMC Myths Dispelled." Accessed February 2, 2017. http://blog.uvahealth.com/2014/11/19/amc-questions-myths-dispelled/.

3. Brigham and Women's Hospital. "Outpatient Surgery." Accessed January 9, 2017. http://healthlibrary.brighamandwomens.org.
4. "How to Choose a Hospital." *Consumer Reports.* Accessed January 9, 2017. http://www.consumerreports.org/cro/2013/01/how-to-choose-a-hospital/index.html.

CHAPTER 3

1. Gail Van Kanegan and Michael Boyette, *How to Survive Your Hospital Stay* (New York: Simon and Schuster, 2003), 12–13.

CHAPTER 4

1. Mayo Clinic. "Personal Health Record: A Tool for Managing Your Health." Accessed January 9, 2017. http://www.mayoclinic.org/healthy-lifestyle/consumer-health/in-depth/personal-health-record/art-20047273.

CHAPTER 5

1. Sharon Theimer, "Headed for the OR? Five Questions to Ask Your Surgeon before the Operation." Mayo Clinic News Network. Accessed January 9, 2017. http://newsnetwork.mayoclinic.org/discussion/headed-for-the-or-mayo-clinic-expert-suggests-5-questions-to-ask-your-surgeon-before-the-operation.
2. American Academy of Orthopaedic Surgeons. "Preparing for Joint Replacement Surgery." Accessed January 9, 2017. http://orthoinfo.aaos.org/topic.cfm?topic=A00220.
3. Theimer.

Chapter 6

1. "Best High Fiber Cereal, Healthful and Tasty." *Consumer Reports.* Accessed January 9, 2017. http://www.consumerreports.org/cro/magazine/2013/09/best-high-fiber-cereal-high-fiber-cereal-cereal-consumer-reports/index.htm.

Chapter 7

1. Agency for Healthcare Research and Quality "20 Tips to Help Prevent Medical Errors: Patient Fact Sheet." Accessed January 9, 2017. https://archive.ahrq.gov/patients-consumers/care-planning/errors/20tips/index.html.
2. Hospital for Special Surgery. "Preventing Urinary Catheter Infections." Accessed January 9, 2017. https://www.hss.edu/quality-preventing-urinary-catheter-infections.asp.
3. M. Pappas, S. Jolly, and S. Vijan. "Defining Appropriate Use of Proton-Pump Inhibitors among Medical Inpatients." *Journal of General Internal Medicine* 31, no. 4 (2016): 364–71.

Chapter 8

1. "Turn Up the Heat: Avoiding Surgical Complications with Adequate Patient Warming." *OR Connection* 6, no. 1 (2011): 14.
2. F. J. Belda, et al. "Supplemental Perioperative Oxygen and the Risk of Surgical Wound Infection: A Randomized Controlled Trial." *Journal of the American Medical Association* 294, no. 16 (2005): 2035–42.
3. Hospital for Special Surgery. "Preventing Blood Clots after Surgery." Accessed October 29, 2016. https://www.hss.edu/quality-preventing-blood-clots.asp.

4. Rebecca Boyle, "FYI: How Does a Drug Get Its Name?" *Popular Science*. Accessed January 9, 2017. http://www.popsci.com/science/article/2013-04/fyi-how-does-drug-get-its-name.

CHAPTER 9

1. American Academy of Orthopaedic Surgeons. "Deep Vein Thrombosis." Accessed January 9, 2017. http://orthoinfo.aaos.org/topic.cfm?topic=A00219.

ABOUT THE AUTHOR

◆ ◆ ◆

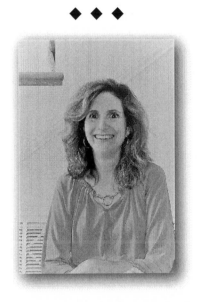

KAYE NEWTON IS AN EXPERIENCED hospital advocate, surgery patient, and caregiver. She lives outside Nashville with her husband, three children, and two dogs.

Made in the USA
Columbia, SC
12 May 2017